$17.96   1-5-00   Lucent   T

Depression

Look for these and other books in the Lucent Overview Series:

Alcoholism
The Brain
Child Abuse
Dealing with Death
Drug Abuse
Eating Disorders
Family Violence
Memory
Mental Illness
Poverty
Suicide

Depression

by Robyn M. Weaver

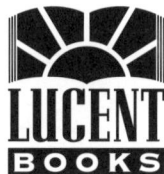

LUCENT
BOOKS

LUCENT *Overview Series*

LUCENT Overview Series

A special thanks to Ann Arnold, Ph.D, and Kathy Foster, Ph.D, both compassionate psychologists, for their unending patience and numerous contributions to the accuracy of this material.

Library of Congress Cataloging-in-Publication Data

Weaver, Robyn.
    Depression / by Robyn M. Weaver.
        p.   cm. — (Lucent overview series)
    Includes bibliographical references and index.
    Summary: Discusses the nature, causes, effects, and treatment of depression, as well as where and how to get help.
    ISBN 1-56006-437-4 (lib.)
    1. Depression, Mental—Juvenile literature.   [1. Depression, Mental.]   I. Title.   II. Series.
RC537.W33   1999
616.85'27—dc21   98-8464
                                                                   CIP
                                                                    AC

*For my mom, in appreciation and honor of
her amazing courage and muscled spirit.*

Contents

Introduction

DEPRESSION IS A disease that affects mind and body. In its most severe form, it can incapacitate the person who is depressed. Some people experience paranoid episodes, such as delusions of being spied on, and these feelings leave them incapable of functioning in society on a day-to-day basis. People with milder forms of depression, who tend not to care about their health or other responsibilities, have trouble eating properly and completing duties at home, work, and school.

Above all else, depression is a disease that leads sufferers to feel isolated and unworthy of help or comfort. In her book *On the Edge of Darkness,* Kathy Cronkite describes the terrible sense of inadequacy she felt before she sought help for her depression:

> I can't figure out where to put the baby down so he is safe, so I'm holding him in one arm while I prepare to bathe him in the kitchen sink. It isn't clean. I can't find any cleanser. I want to cry. I am a terrible mother because I can't bathe the baby. I am a terrible housewife because I can't find the cleanser. I am a terrible household manager, because maybe there isn't any cleanser.[1]

Depression in all its various forms—from mild to severe—is thought to afflict a million Americans every year. Despite its relatively common occurrence, depression has long been misunderstood. Even in recent times, going back only fifty to sixty years, depression was generally viewed as a personal failing, not as a condition for which physical causes might be sought.

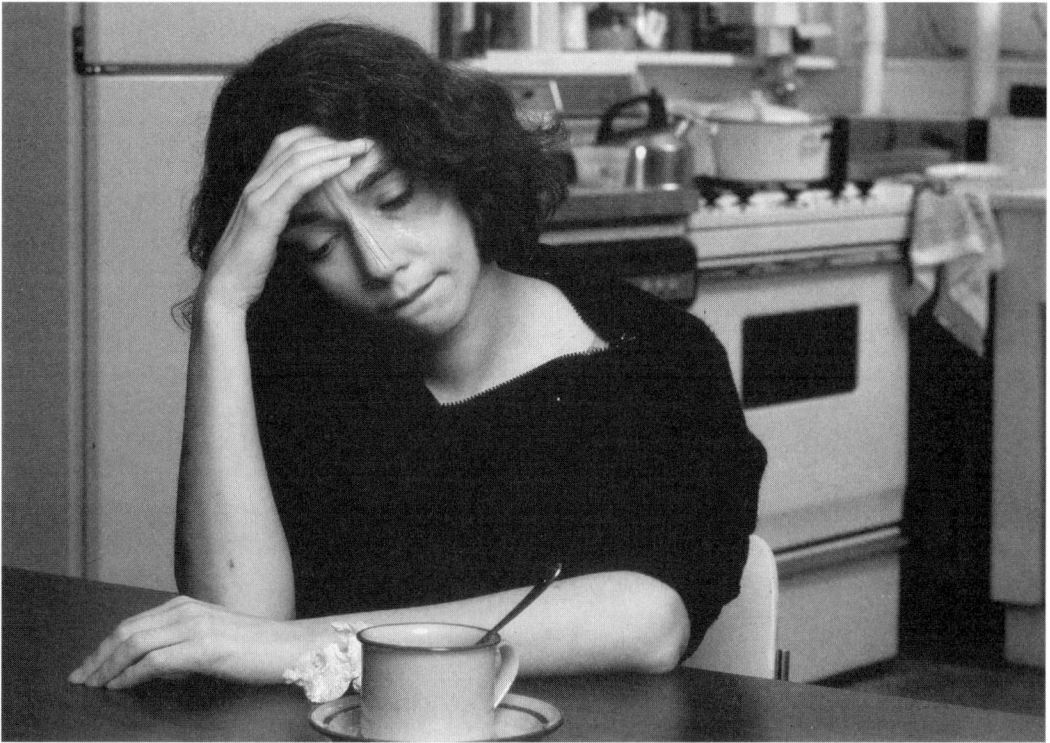

A woman suffers from the effects of depression. Depression may affect more than a million Americans a year.

This lack of understanding in the recent past may be explained by the rather primitive methods then available for studying diseases brought on by abnormalities in body chemistry. Unfortunately, misconceptions persist today, even as new information emerges about the causes of depression and methods for treating it. To the uninformed, including those who have experienced their own depression or the illness of a close friend or relative, the symptoms of depression can be confusing, frightening, and sometimes even bizarre.

Behavior may change in seemingly unexplainable ways. Normally energetic people may start oversleeping. Normally diet-wise people may start eating too much or too little. Cheerful people have been known to start expressing gloomy thoughts, such as "Nothing ever goes right for me anymore." People suffering from the severest form of depression experience suicidal thoughts; if this happens, immediate help is needed.

Those who seek help will learn, as will their friends and relatives, that depressed behavior stems not from insanity or a flawed personality, but from a biochemical imbalance that can be corrected if properly diagnosed and treated. They will also learn that stressful events, and their own ways of coping with stress, may trigger the chemical changes that bring on depressive episodes. Sometimes the answer to these problems can be found in prescribed drugs or counseling. And sometimes both these treatment modes are required, or a combination of them with additional alternative therapies.

Even with the greater knowledge available today about the causes and treatment of depression, many people have trouble seeing past the odd behaviors associated with the disease. In fact, many friends, coworkers, and relatives are so uncomfortable with the symptoms of depression that they discourage sufferers from talking about it.

Rod Steiger, an Academy Award–winning actor who has battled depression, would like more people to know how common the disease is. He suspects, however, that his frankness has alarmed financial powers in the entertainment business to the extent of hurting his career:

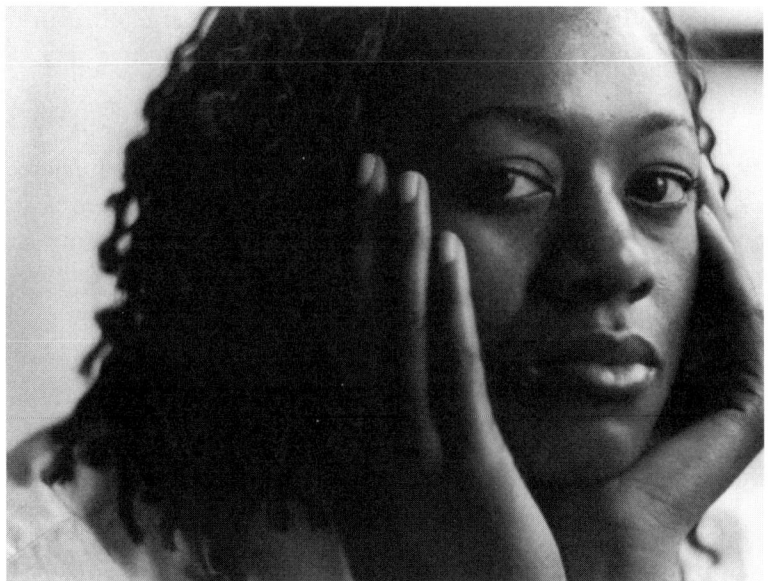

Depression can lead to a feeling of hopelessness and, if left untreated, to suicide.

I have been opening my mouth in newspaper interviews since I've been feeling better the past three years, and businesspeople around me are quite hysterical. It might have damaged me to some degree in the profession. I don't know. Across the country, one in five has a mental disease. It's about time we began to talk about this thing.[2]

When depressive episodes become more frequent and treatment is not given, hopelessness can set in. And indeed, one of the greatest threats facing people who become depressed, especially those who do not obtain treatment, is suicide. Jan Fawcett, an expert on depression, alcoholism, and well-being, estimates that 93 to 95 percent of people who committed suicide were experiencing a psychiatric illness, most commonly depression.

Today, it is believed that people who suffer from depression also develop secondary abuse problems such as alcoholism and drug addiction. These harmful behaviors represent the individuals' misguided attempts to dull the negative feelings that accompany depression. Researchers think the eating disorders anorexia and bulimia also are indications of feelings of low self-worth and hopelessness. Recent studies link these disorders with depressive illness.

Despite new information about depression, and despite a high success rate of treatment, depression remains shrouded in mystery and confusion. More than anything, people need to learn that they can encourage their loved ones to manage and overcome depression, just as if they were helping them live with heart disease. Sometimes the greatest support is found in simple words like "I care about you. Let's go find someone to help."

1

About Depression

WINSTON CHURCHILL CALLED it his black dog. And although a trusted physician diagnosed Britain's great leader with depression, no one was ever able to convince Churchill to seek professional help. In the 1930s, to participate in sessions with a psychiatrist or to receive the common treatment, electric shock therapy, would have been political suicide. The stigma of mental illness in the early decades of this century was indeed a reality, and depression was socially unacceptable. People didn't talk about it, except to repeat the conventional wisdom of the day—that the depressed were unworthy and weak-willed persons.

Even today, depression sufferers believe society needs help accepting the disease as a biochemical imbalance. Mike Wallace, well-respected journalist, has this to say about his own depression:

> People who don't know, who say it's self-indulgence, sound callous, but it's not callousness born of indifference; I think it's callousness born of ignorance. That kind of ignorance we've got to get rid of.[3]

What is it?

Depression is a physical illness. It results from a biochemical imbalance in the brain that affects the whole body, not just the brain or its thought patterns. Depression comes in different forms. One of the most common forms is unipolar disorder, more often called major depression. A more severe form, classified as bipolar disorder, was formerly known as manic depression. A third form, dysthymia, is a long-lasting, low-level depression, but not as common as the other two forms.

Each year over $30 billion is spent on diagnosing and treating depression in all its many forms, yet only one in three people who suffer from this illness seeks treatment. With advanced medical knowledge readily available, it is perhaps surprising that so few people ask for help.

One reason lies in the very nature of the disease. Because early signs of depression are subtle, often no more than periods of low energy or pessimistic thinking, most people feel they can handle the temporary "down" phase on their own. If help is not obtained, however, harmful behaviors may emerge. Some depressed people quit eating, while others eat too much, trying to distract themselves and avoid their emotional discomfort. Many depressed people simply won't get out of bed. In other forms of depression, physical symptoms such as chest pains, severe headaches, or stomach disorders will escalate to the point of causing concern among friends and family members.

A counselor works with a man suffering from depression. Many depressed people refuse to seek help because they fear the stigma of mental illness.

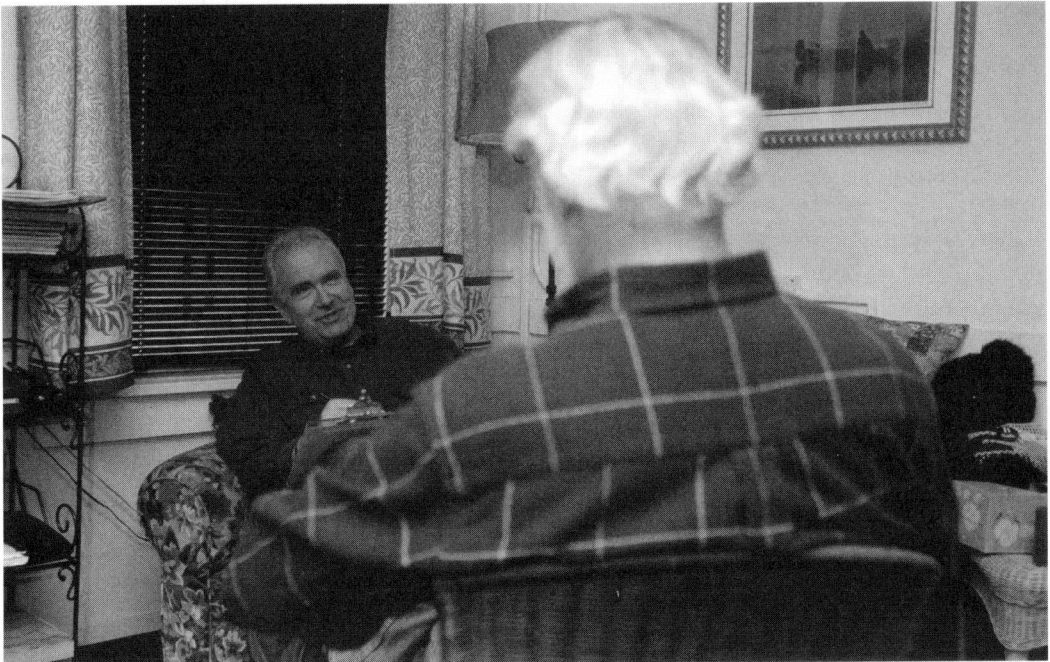

Unfortunately, these caring people, the sufferer's first-line support system, often fail to identify the symptoms of depression. Thus they are unable to steer their loved ones down the road to better health. The onset of symptoms severe enough to distress family and friends is a crucial stage. It is dangerous as well, for often depression fogs the sufferer's mind so badly that he or she does not see the need to get help, or imagines that suicide is the only solution. Even with today's clearer picture of depression and its improved treatment therapies, 15 percent of all people who are tormented with bouts of depression end their lives.

David Hughes, an engineer for Lockheed-Martin, suffered through episodes of depression as a teen. Before he graduated from high school he underwent stomach surgery to relieve an ulcer. Later, in his mid-twenties, his wife left him after only three years of marriage, and the rejection threw Hughes into a black hole of depression that lasted for months. Despite encouraging words and support from

Friends and family members may not realize that someone they care about is depressed.

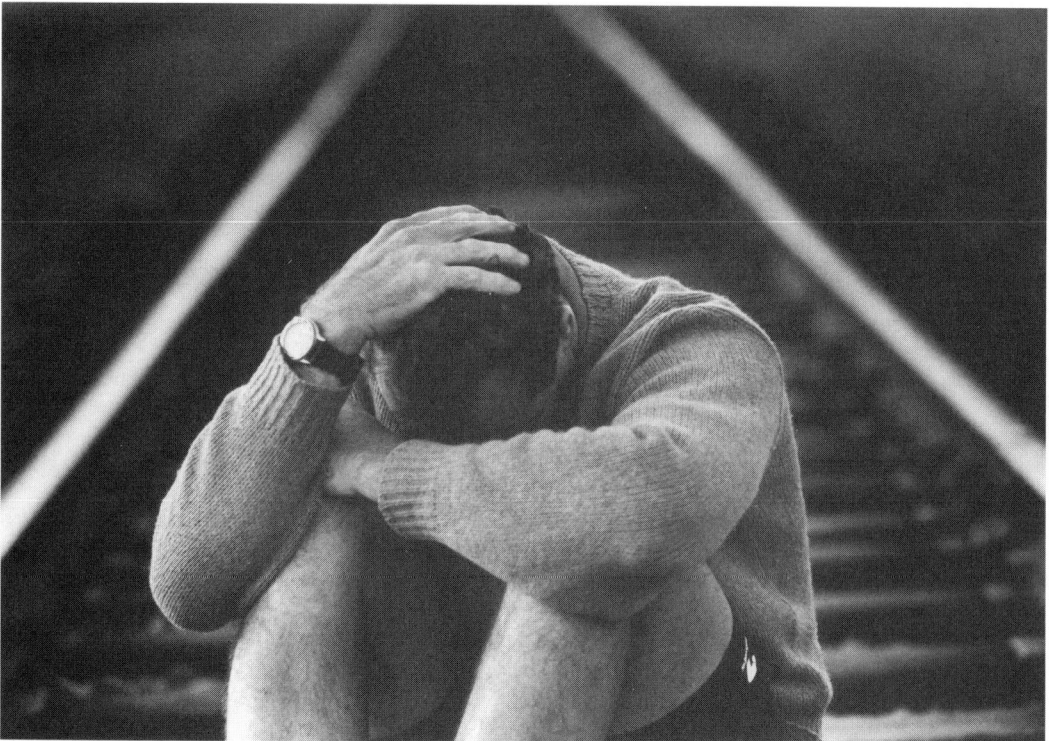

friends, he couldn't rid himself of the terrible despair. To escape those feelings of hopelessness and failure, he began entertaining thoughts of suicide:

> My lack of self-confidence became so bad I actually lost my voice. My bosses sent me to one doctor after another until I finally had to face the fact my physical problem was related to what was going on in my brain.

> At first I thought, "God, just take me home. I'm tired of all these horrible feelings." But then, I checked myself into a day treatment center for a couple of weeks and I was diagnosed right away with major depression.

> They gave me some medication that worked pretty well, and the talks with my therapist really helped a lot. She showed me different thinking processes, which will help with my stress level, and referred me to a speech therapist, who is helping me regain my voice.[4]

Symptoms of major depression

David Hughes did not seek help until his illness had become so noticeable at work that a supervisor forced the issue. The chronic hoarseness hampered Hughes's job capabilities so severely that he was at risk of losing his job.

Although a raspy voice is not a common symptom of major depression, the underlying low self-esteem that plagued Hughes is nearly always found. Other symptoms of major depression include feelings of hopelessness or unworthiness. Some people simply can't overcome a persistent sad or "empty" feeling, while others are constantly negative, pessimistic, or irritable. Other clues may signal depression, as well: difficulty in concentrating, for example, or problems with remembering or making decisions. The more obvious symptoms—bouts of crying or suicidal thoughts and actions—are generally reliable behavioral signs of depression.

Other symptoms that sometimes accompany depression include sleep disturbances, such as insomnia or oversleeping. A decrease in pleasurable activities (including sex), as well as chronic headaches, pains, or digestive problems that fail to respond to treatment, have all been noted as precursors of depression.

The Symptoms of Clinical Depression

According to the American Psychiatric Association, clinical depression can be diagnosed when someone exhibits five or more of the following symptoms (not related to any medical condition or drugs) during a two-week period:

▶ a depressed mood most of the day, nearly every day

▶ markedly diminished interest or pleasure in most activity during the day, nearly every day

▶ significant weight loss or gain over a month (for instance, a change of more than 5 percent of body weight)

▶ significant change in sleep habits—sleeping far more or far less than usual

▶ extreme agitation or extreme slowness of movement nearly every day

▶ fatigue or loss of energy nearly every day

▶ feelings of worthlessness or excessive guilt every day

▶ diminished ability to concentrate, or indecisiveness nearly every day

▶ recurrent thoughts of death or suicide (or suicide attempts)

Almost everyone can claim a few of those symptoms at any given time, especially during times of great stress. Periods of grief, sadness, or disappointment, often referred to as feeling "blue" or "down in the dumps," occur naturally after many life events—a physical trauma, for example, or the death of a loved one, a divorce, or a job transition. Mental health professionals recognize these episodes as normal "life adjustment" phases, during which symptoms such as sleep disturbances typically show up for a short time.

However, a person who has several symptoms that persist or increase in severity over a few weeks or months most likely needs professional help. A professional can determine the severity of depression, whether it requires treatment, and if so, what form it should take.

Symptoms of bipolar disorder

Probably the most severe form of depression is bipolar disorder, also still known in the popular press as manic

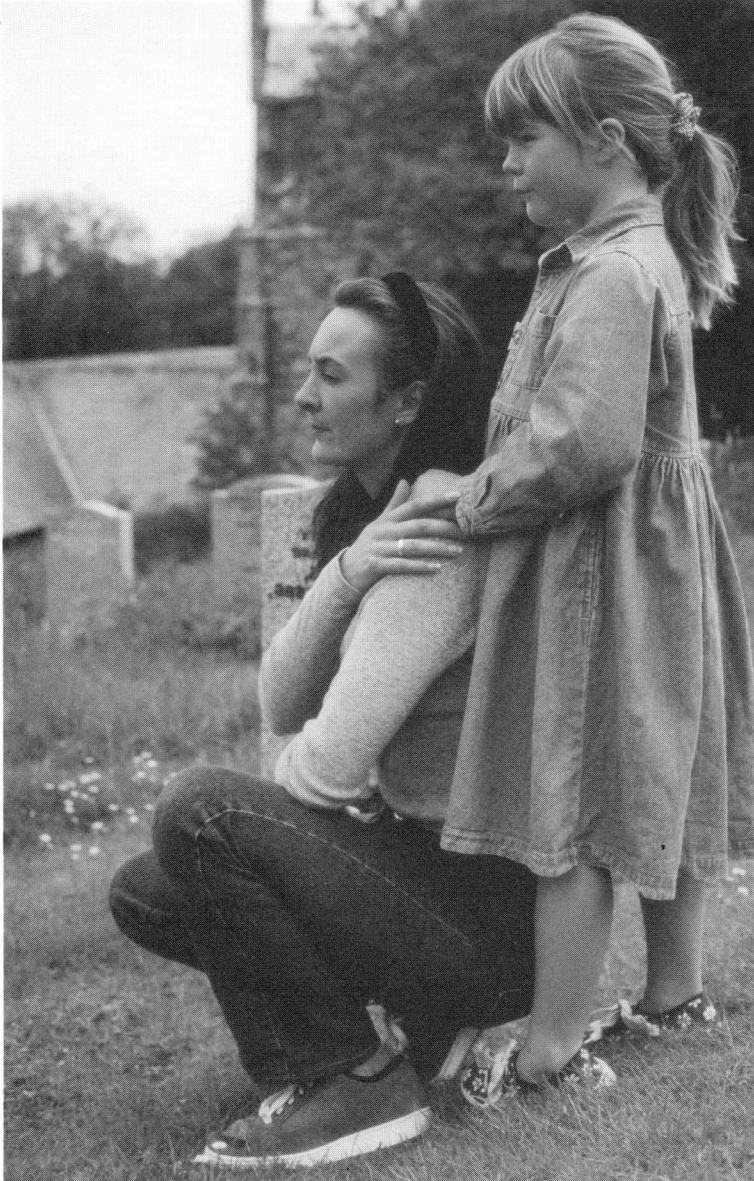

A woman and her daughter visit the grave of a loved one. Stressful events such as the death of a family member may cause temporary depression. Depressed feelings that persist may be a sign of illness.

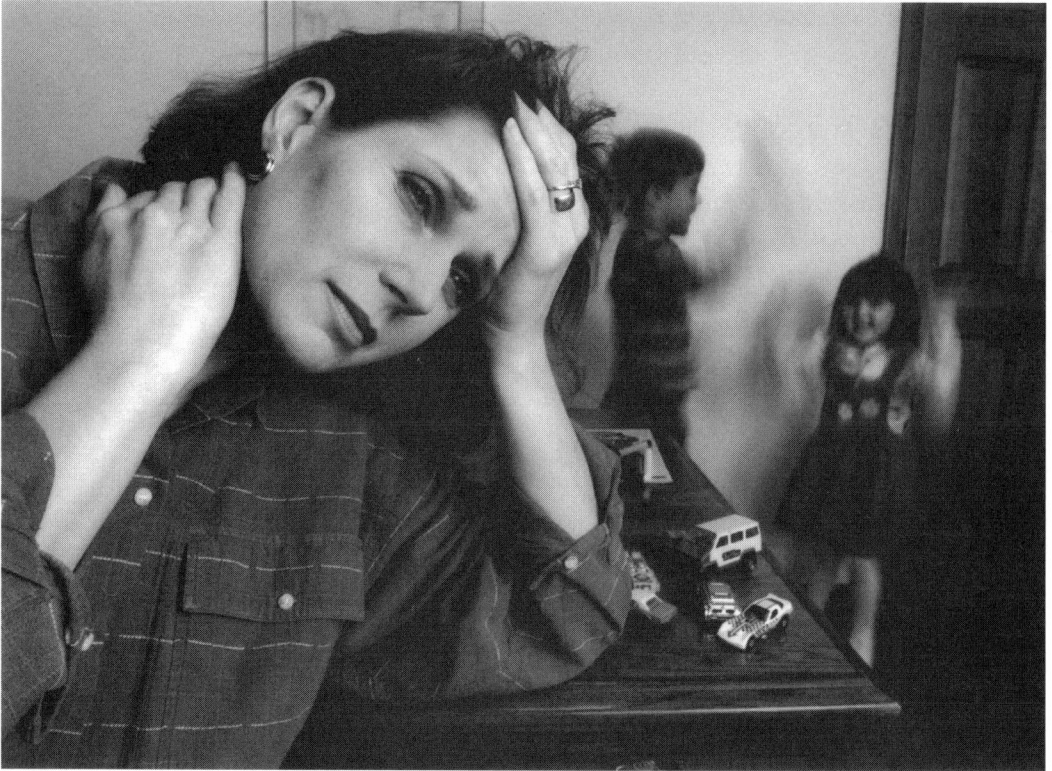

The extreme highs and lows of bipolar disorder may strain family relationships.

depression. Many of its symptoms overlap those of unipolar disorder; only qualified professionals can properly distinguish between the two illnesses.

People prone to bipolar disorder may develop more pronounced symptoms of the excited, almost euphoric feeling called mania. Some experience delusions or hallucinations when in these "high" moods. They have an increased energy level and suddenly begin to talk too fast, move in quicker steps, and indulge in promiscuous sexual activity. Their thoughts tend to race together, and they believe everything they see or feel centers around them. These people are easily distracted and claim to need only a few hours of sleep a night.

Bipolar disorder sufferers often find their symptoms highly discouraging, disabling, and disrupting over a period of years. More than two million people with bipolar disorder experience the terrible "lows," or periods of exhaustion and overwhelming hopelessness over their inability to control the manic periods.

In April 1997, *Good Housekeeping* magazine featured the story of a woman named Faye Shannon, who revealed some of the horrors she had experienced as a "manic depressive." Although Shannon believes her condition was brought on by a series of stressing circumstances, her first bout of paranoia was triggered by an ordinary occurrence.

> One morning I spent two hours frantically searching for my car keys. I was furious at George [her husband], convinced he must have moved them—until I found the keys exactly where I left them. At work that same day, I was overwhelmed by feelings of sadness and sat frozen at my desk. When a woman shared a bit of office gossip, I laughed hysterically . . . soon after, I became convinced that our office was bugged. . . . Then I began having delusions involving the FBI. Suddenly I *knew* I was wanted on a top-secret project.[5]

Shannon's behavior and thinking patterns reflect the manic "highs" of bipolar disorder. Later in the article she tells of feeling so tired she could barely get out of bed to care for her small children: these experiences represent the numbing "lows" of the disorder.

Symptoms of dysthymia

A third form of depression, dysthymia, is often referred to as mild, but chronic depression. It has been estimated that 5 to 15 percent of all patients in a family doctor's office have dysthymia, a condition that is more commonly diagnosed in women than in men.

To be diagnosed with this form of depression, a person must have several symptoms over a two-year period. Often these include low self-esteem, difficulty concentrating, withdrawal, pessimism, and hopelessness.

Constant tiredness, another possible symptom, was what sent one man, himself a psychologist, to a physician for help: "My problem with dysthymia was characterized by fatigue . . . by the afternoon, I became very tired and less clear in my thinking; I had to take a nap every afternoon or I couldn't work in the evening."[6] The doctor prescribed the antidepressant Elavil, and the patient improved significantly.

A woman, now happy with life and living in New York, had suffered through twelve years of feeling glum and down. One day she happened to see a television program that defined depression in terms of all the symptoms she thought were just part of her personality. She sought treatment for her dysthymia, and today her life has changed for the better.

Many other people who experience prolonged "blue" periods, which are neither alarming nor bizarre, also tend to assume that they are just prone to feeling bad. John C. Markowitz, an associate professor of clinical psychiatry at Cornell University Medical College says, "Dysthymia causes you to think there's something wrong with your character."[7]

People with dysthymia need to be reassured that they are not walking examples of character defects, even when other people criticize them for "not trying hard enough." For example, it is normal for a dysthymic person not to care about appearance, or about having fun, or about eating properly. These symptoms may seem minor, but experts believe that people who undergo periods of dysthymia are more likely to experience episodes of major depression later in their lives.

Depression and other illnesses

No matter what form depression takes, its victims have a hard time looking after their physical health. People who are not thinking clearly, a category that includes many depression sufferers, often neglect their bodily health. They also may start drinking too much, taking drugs, or experimenting with other destructive behaviors as they try to be happier or to lose their feelings of emptiness. According to a recent study, some form of substance abuse or drug dependence is found in nearly one out of three depressed people (32%).

Depression is also common in people diagnosed with cancer, stroke, diabetes, and other chronic medical conditions. The hopelessness and helplessness that often accompany such diagnoses can affect a patient's thinking patterns, and treating depression, when it appears, can have a positive effect on the course of these other illnesses. For example, people who are unable to concentrate because of depression cannot properly manage the medications or diet needed to maintain their blood pressure or insulin level in the prescribed range. The importance of

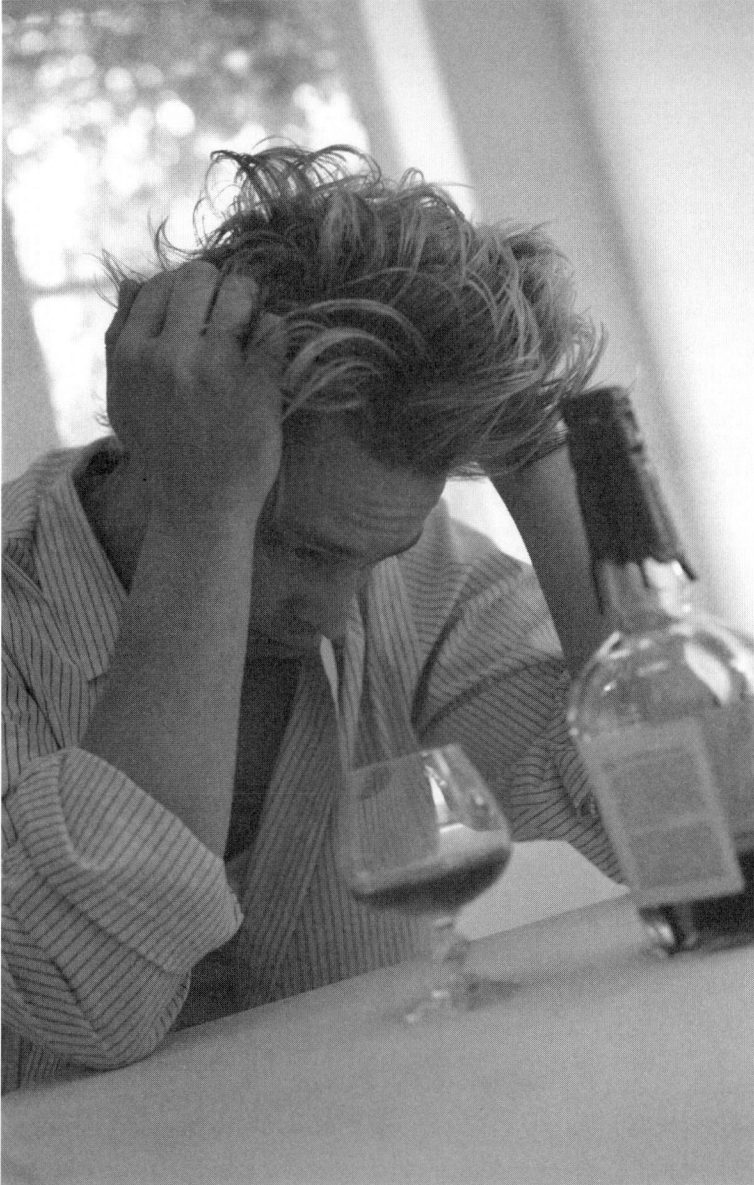

One-third of all people experiencing depression turn to alcohol or drugs to escape their feelings. Such self-destructive behavior may prevent a depressed person from seeking help.

diagnosing depression so these people can participate effectively in their own treatment is slowly gaining acceptance both in the medical communities and in society at large.

The more people understand about depression, the more likely it is to be recognized and diagnosed. A greater rate of diagnosis will ease both physical and mental discomfort to the patient, and will lessen the distress of friends and family members who want to help.

2

What Causes Depression?

DESPITE NUMEROUS CASE studies and break-throughs in genetic research, the exact cause of depression is still hard to pinpoint. However, a high number of studies conclude that depressive disorders have a biological basis and are more common in people with certain biochemical makeups. This is a great advance over the perspective of the recent past, when depression was attributed to a patient's lifestyle, or said to result solely from psychological problems following a traumatic or stressful event.

Many mental health professionals today believe that depression results from a combination of biochemical and psychological factors. For example, an event such as the death of a family member might be sufficiently traumatic to trigger an imbalance of chemicals in the brain. This imbalance, in turn, might result in depression curable only by the same or other chemicals. These chemicals may be stimulated naturally by means of a growing array of therapies, or they may be administered in the form of prescription drugs.

Researchers are also investigating the possibility that heredity, or the genetic makeup people receive from their parents, plays a role in depression. Although efforts to identify the causes of depression continue, most experts no longer believe that environment and lifestyle are solely responsible.

24

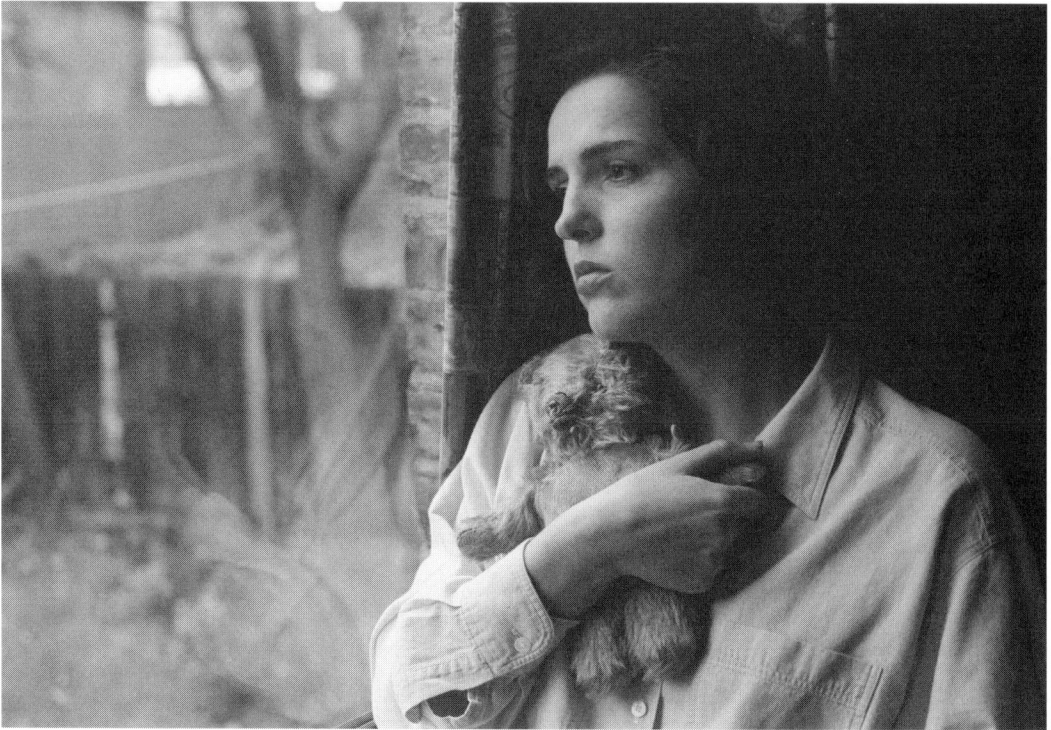

Depression often produces feelings of isolation and loneliness. Doctors today believe that hereditary and biochemical factors are involved in depression.

Chemical messengers

Both major depression and mania have been linked with improper functioning of certain neurotransmitters, or chemical messengers, in the brain. These chemical messengers transmit signals from one nerve cell to another across the spaces between cells, called synapses. The signals set into motion interactions that induce people to behave, feel, or think in certain ways. That's why people with depression often display "behavior" symptoms, such as overeating, rather than "physical" symptoms, such as a high temperature.

Today it is widely believed that a shortage of certain neurotransmitters can cause depression. Studies have shown that three neurotransmitters—norepinephrine, serotonin, and dopamine—are greatly reduced or missing in people diagnosed with depression. Low serotonin has also been linked to the number-one cause of death among depression sufferers: researchers have discovered lower levels of serotonin in certain areas of the brains of people who committed suicide than in the brains of people who have died from other causes. Since the presence of serotonin in these areas is believed to discourage violent actions, people with *too little* serotonin might experience abnormally high suicidal or aggressive feelings.

Hormone imbalance

Another possible biological source of depression lies in the endocrine system, the glands, such as the thyroid gland, that regulate hormones in the body. Hormones are the compounds that stimulate the body to perform proper growth, digestion, and other necessary functions.

Irregularities in hormonal compounds can cause mood disorder symptoms. For example, hypothyroidism, the result of a sluggish thyroid gland, can also bring about a mental numbness, as seen in people who lose interest in daily tasks. And hyperthyroidism, the result of an overactive thyroid, can bring about symptoms of mania, with excessive energy and restlessness. Correcting such hormone imbalances can eliminate some troubling behavioral symptoms.

Genetics

Hereditary factors may also play a role in determining who is at risk of developing a depressive disorder. It has been known for much of this century that children inherit physical characteristics from each parent. For example, one baby might inherit his father's bone structure; another might have eyes like her mother's. These traits are transmitted by units of inheritance called genes, and tiny molecules in human genes also hold clues to the biological basis of depression. Research now suggests that children can also inherit a tendency to develop depression. Such a tendency is called genetic predisposition.

Missing cells

Missing brain cells offer another substantial clue to the biological causes of depression. Dr. Wayne Drevets, a researcher at the University of Pittsburgh, recently analyzed samples of brain tissue from people diagnosed with depression. He and his fellow researchers discovered that glial cells, which are essential in providing serotonin to the brain, were completely absent or present only in low numbers. "We were stunned," Drevets said. "We think this is the single most important finding in mood disorders."[8] In

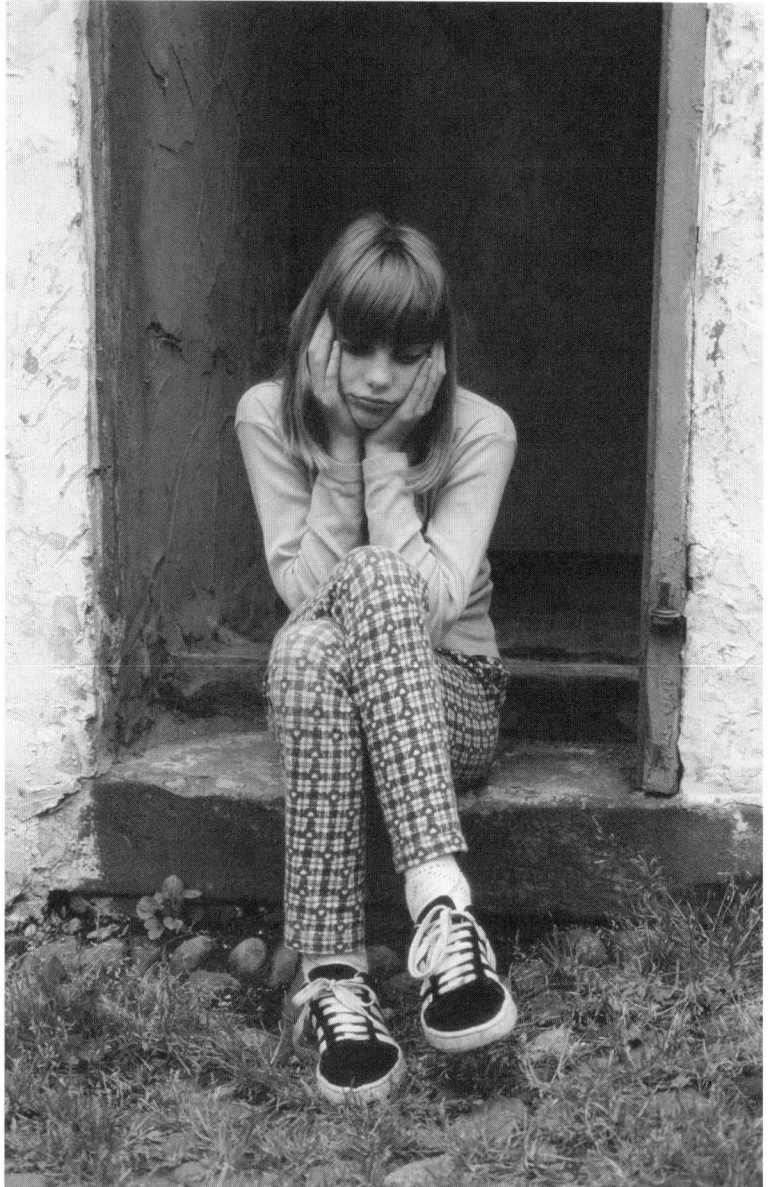

Young people who experience depression may have inherited the condition from their parents.

confirming the absence of the cells that supply serotonin to the brain, Drevets and his team have narrowed the search for the biological causes of depression.

Vitamin deficiencies

The biochemical imbalances that lead to depression may include vitamin deficiencies. For example, the B vitamins are important in brain metabolism, brain growth, and proper mental function. If brain function is hindered because the body does not receive enough B vitamins, depression may result.

During the early 1930s, in the southern United States, two hundred thousand victims of the disease called pellagra ended up in mental hospitals, suffering from depression, intellectual impairment, stomach problems, and skin eruptions. Research discovered a lack of vitamin B_3, also known as niacin, in these patients' diets. After the widespread outbreak, niacin was added to most commercial cereal products and pellagra vanished from industrialized countries; it remains prevalent in less developed regions of the world.

The long-ago experience with pellagra led researchers to suspect other vitamin deficiencies as causes for depression. Thus is was not surprising when, in 1982, a study confirmed that over half of 127 patients admitted into a British general hospital psychiatric unit were deficient in at least one B vitamin. And with the discovery that low levels of certain B vitamins are common in people suffering from the disease, research on B vitamins and their relationship to depression has attracted considerable attention.

One doctor tells of a forty-seven-year-old woman who reported seeing UFOs and announced that Jesus had commanded her to board one of them. Her concerned family took her to the hospital, where doctors noticed that the patient looked older than her recorded age. Family members described the woman as having become sad, tired, and reclusive. When a severe deficiency of vitamin B_{12} was discovered, and treated, the patient no longer saw spaceships and was restored to health.

Shortages of B_{12} can cause some symptoms of depression. Because this vitamin is found in meat and in other animal proteins such as milk and cheese, strict vegetarians sometimes exhibit mood changes, paranoia, irritability, confusion, and hallucinations. If in fact B_{12} deficiency is the only cause of the symptoms, taking vitamin supplements can help to alleviate these characteristics of depression.

Other B vitamins that contribute to the body's mental health are folic acid, B_6 (pyridoxine), B_2 (riboflavin), and B_1 (thiamine). A person who has a shortage of these crucial vitamins will suffer emotionally as well as physically.

Psychological factors

Although researchers now believe that the primary agents of depression are biochemical, stress due to psychological factors can cause changes in the body chemistry. It is these changes that are thought to create the biochemical imbalances that disrupt proper brain functions.

Early theories about depression, however, were dominated by the ideas of Sigmund Freud, considered the founder of psychoanalysis (the study of thinking processes). Freud believed that depression was the product of unexpressed and unconscious rage that developed as a reaction to feeling helpless or being dependent on others. A traumatic event, such as the loss of a loved one or even the arrival of a new baby, could trigger feelings of helplessness and dependence and lead to a sense of abandonment. According to Freud, the arrival of a new baby, for example, could create in an older child overwhelming feelings of being abandoned.

Freud's theories center on the psychological bind of a child in such a situation. He or she cannot express rage directly, for this might anger the mother. But the only alternative is to swallow the feelings, to keep the anger and loss inside; and this route produces depression. As the child grows, this reaction to losses becomes habitual, a learned response, and depression occurs again and again, sometimes with greater intensity.

The learned response theory is compatible with the altered brain chemical theory that is more common today. Both theories state that continued negativity can set in motion certain biochemical patterns that may lead to depression. Levels of stress present in an individual's environment can increase or decrease the chemical balance and affect those patterns.

To learn about particular thought patterns, mental health professionals use the Social Readjustment Scale, a tool for charting stress levels. The scale assigns numerical values to a number of stress-inducing life events. The person whose stress level is to be measured checks off all the events that apply to his or her recent life, and the person administering the test notes the scale's value for each event selected. These values are added up and averaged; the result is a number indicating the person's stress level.

Developed in 1960 by Thomas Holmes and Richard Rache as a means of determining general health and potential risk of illness, the Social Readjustment Scale is used

A young girl views her newborn sibling. Early psychoanalysts such as Sigmund Freud believed events such as the birth of a sibling triggered feelings of rage and abandonment.

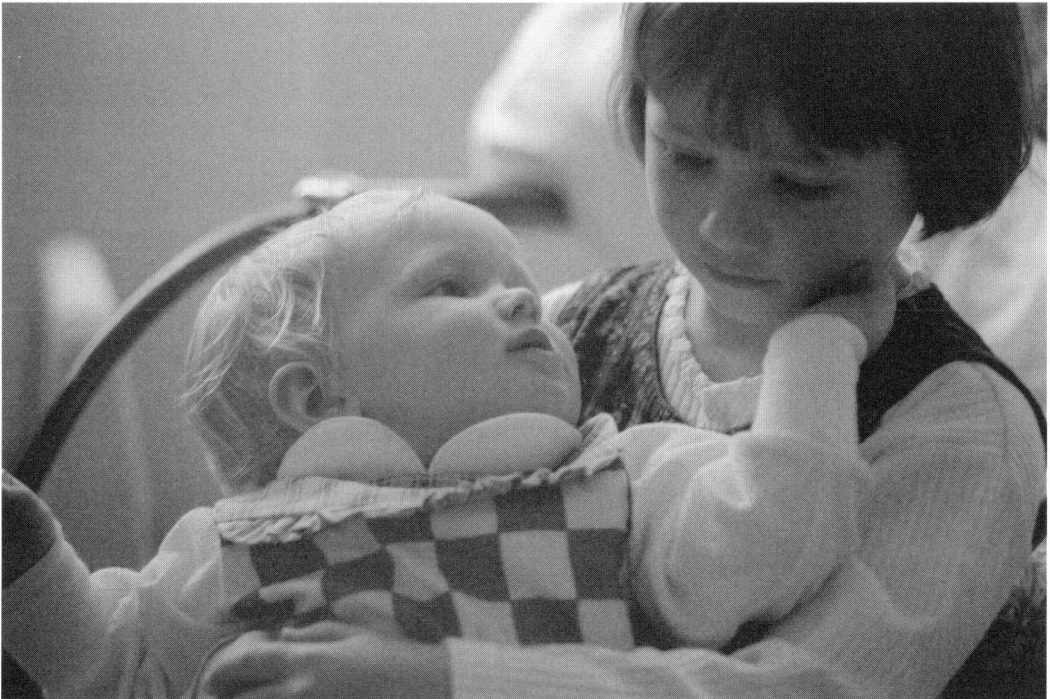

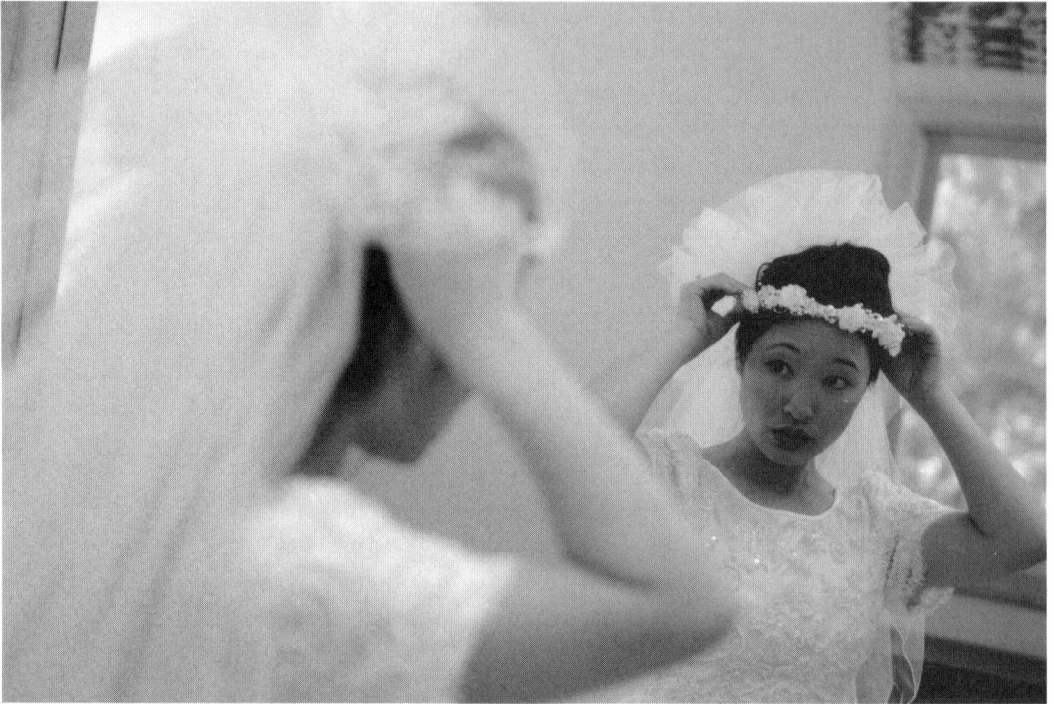

A young woman adjusts her veil. An event such as a wedding, that creates stress and high expectations of happiness, may trigger bouts of depression.

frequently today by mental health professionals for weighing the risk of depressive disorders in their patients or clients.

For example, the death of a spouse, the highest rated level of stress, is given a value of 100. Divorce is next, with a value of 73. Marital separation, jail terms, and deaths of close family members are given values in the 60s.

Some might think that only negative life events cause unhealthy stress, but getting married pulls a 50-point value, indicating that even "good" things can alter the biochemical processes that occur in the brain. Similarly, applying for and taking out a loan might represent an exciting start toward a new house, but the underlying responsibilities could trigger a severe stress chain reaction.

Psychiatrist Alan Romanoski, at Johns Hopkins University, concluded from data on eight hundred people that 86 percent of major depressions are diagnosed shortly after a real-life stressful event or situation. This is a strong statement in support of the contention that psychological factors can trigger the biochemical imbalances that lead to depression, no less than deficiencies of essential vitamins and hormones, or genetic predisposition.

These latest insights encourage scientists to continue research that teaches them more about the causes of depression. Consequently, greater public awareness should increase the quality of life for those who suffer from depressive disorders. By the same token, the understanding that depression is a disease, not a character defect, should result in more compassionate treatment of depressed people in their daily lives.

3

Those at Risk

Most EXPERTS AGREE that depression develops because of biochemical changes in a person's body. Now researchers wanted to know whether any specific groups of people are at higher risk. First the investigators reviewed the causes of depression. Then they studied groups that included people who had suffered the severe stresses believed to cause the biochemical imbalances that lead to depression. They also included representatives of groups whose body chemistry naturally alters during the course of their lives.

These studies suggest that four main risk groups exist: people who have experienced extreme abuse; women, whose body chemistry naturally alters throughout their lives; the elderly; and children.

Abuse victims

Extreme stress is one of the biggest catalysts of depression. People who have experienced abuse—whether physical, sexual, or emotional—often develop the symptoms of depression. The frightening, degrading physical or mental battering they receive commonly chips away at their self-esteem and causes them to feel extremely negative about themselves. Experts believe that these abnormally harsh feelings alter the balance of chemicals in the brain, leading to depression.

Experience bears this out. Family therapist Kathryn Foster, Ph.D., has counseled many abuse victims. In her practice, she has often found that people who were abused later develop depression:

Almost all of the abuse victims I work with suffer from some sort of depressive disorder. When abuse is internalized, it makes for very negative self-talk and all that negativity causes chemical changes in the brain.[9]

Negative thinking patterns, which are a typical response to abuse, are also known as "learned helplessness." This term means that people who grow up exposed to bad attitudes about work, family members, or other activities tend

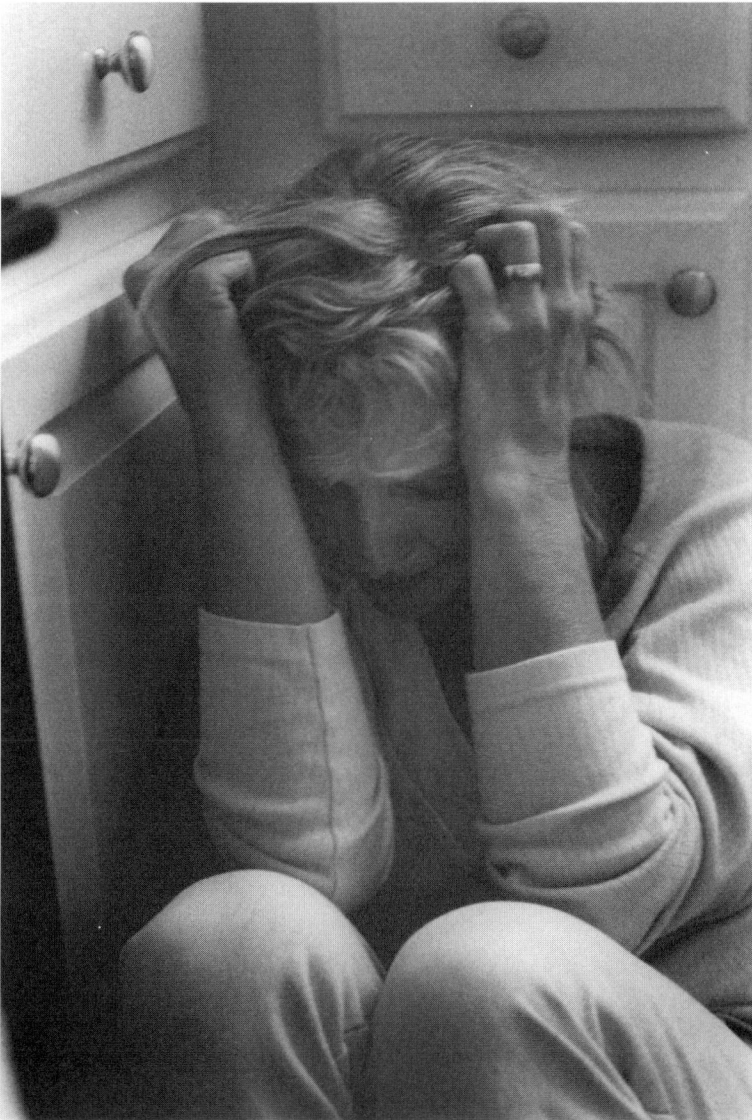

A victim of domestic violence cowers in the kitchen. Abuse victims or others who experience extreme and constant stress often suffer from depression.

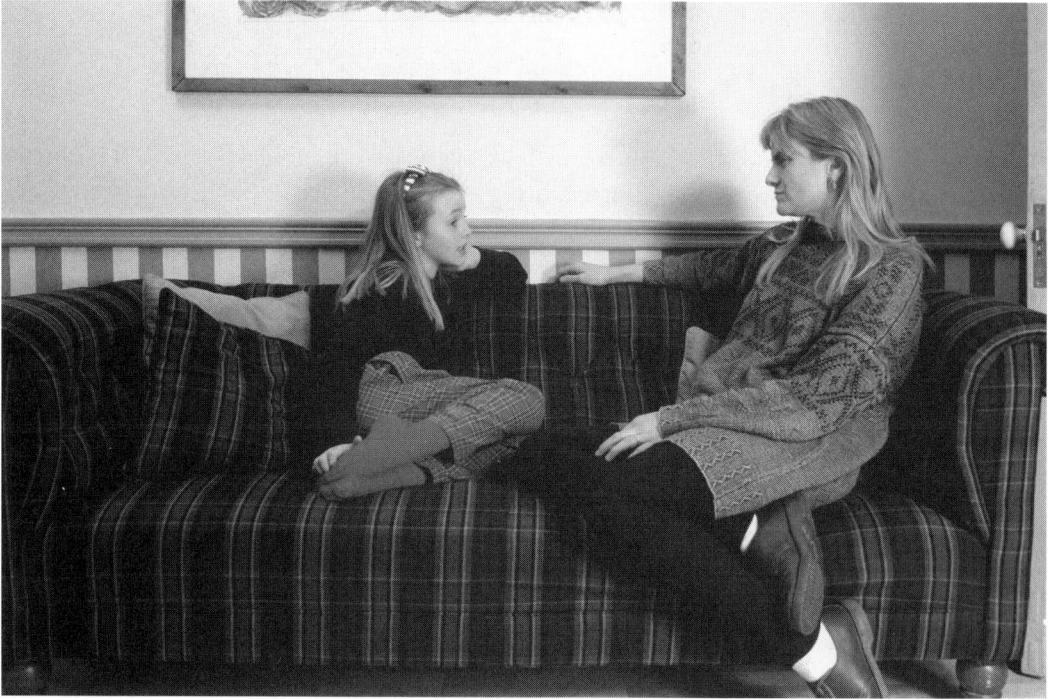

Parents who talk to their children about stressful events such as divorce or a death in the family can significantly reduce the child's stress level and thus alleviate feelings of hopelessness, guilt, and depression.

to recycle those very attitudes. When these people are faced with a rough life event, such as loss of a job, their stress levels jump.

Psychologists refer to these thinking patterns as explanatory styles or attribution styles. Martin Seligman, director of clinical training at the University of Pennsylvania, Philadelphia, says people learn to feel helpless by the way they explain things to themselves. Thus children who come to believe that they are to blame for all the bad things that happen to them build layers and layers of stressful thinking. If no one intervenes to explain that most undesirable events—a divorce, a hurricane, the death of a pet—are beyond a child's control, such children, like abuse victims, will run a higher risk of developing depression as teens or adults.

Women

Women constitute another high-risk group for developing depression. Depression is diagnosed almost twice as

often in women as in men. This 2:1 ratio holds true regardless of racial or ethnic background and regardless of economic or social status. Some experts believe that the number of men suffering from depression is underreported because men are less likely to seek help and obtain a diagnosis. One important factor, however, that may account for higher levels of depression in women: the normal hormone changes women experience at various stages in their lives.

The first phase of intense hormone changes females face begins during their early teen years. With the onset of menstruation, hormone levels vary constantly, and these levels can affect mood and behavior. Dr. Mark S. Gold, in his book *Good News About Depression,* reports:

> We know that women's suicide attempts and threats, as well as their admissions to psychiatric hospitals, increase premenstrually. We know that over two-thirds of women with a history of severe depression have significant premenstrual lows. We know, too, that women with premenstrual mood problems are likely to have a family history of depression.[10]

Premenstrual syndrome, also known as PMS, affects many women in the few days before menstruation begins;

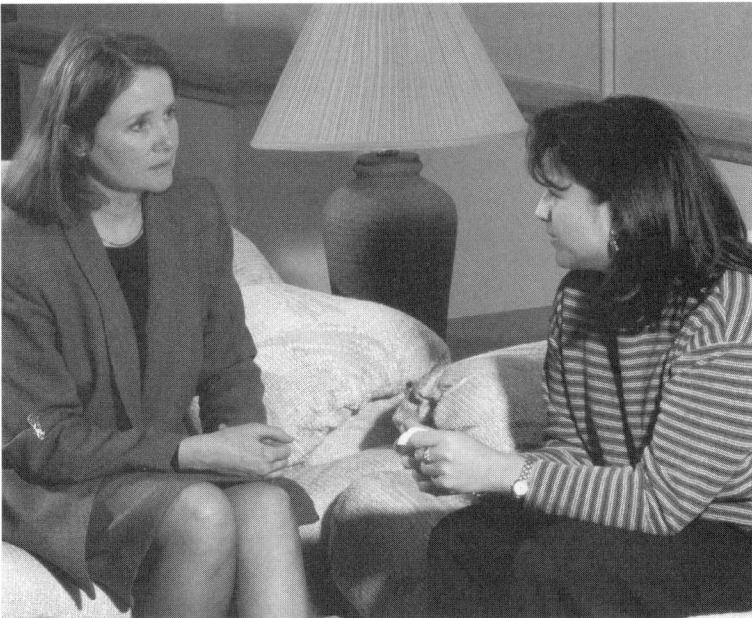

A depressed woman seeks help from a therapist. Women are more likely to suffer from depression than men. They are also more likely to seek help.

symptoms include bloating, irritability, and headaches. For women with depression, however, these symptoms and possibly others may be magnified during the normal premenstrual changes in hormonal levels.

The characteristic mood swings of PMS, and the accompanying erratic behaviors, such as yelling and crying, have encouraged studies to determine whether PMS is strongly related to other depressive orders. The exaggerated behaviors of PMS and the hormonal imbalances that naturally precede menstruation certainly point to a connection to depression.

Perhaps the most common times for women to feel depressed come during pregnancy and in the postpartum period, the week or so after giving birth. The obvious physical changes of pregnancy are paralleled internally by changes in a woman's hormones. When the hormones change, so do women's moods. Some women become more emotionally sensitive. Their feelings are easily hurt. Some women experience a higher level of anxiety, and they become grumpy or intolerant when dealing with friends, family, and coworkers.

Immediately after delivering a baby, a woman continues to experience hormone changes, sometimes for several days. Dr. Gold says, "The vast majority of women endure 'maternity blues' which in its mildest form affects 70–80 percent of all women following the birth of a child."[11] Some of these women feel a lingering sadness, along with a reduced energy level. However, most new mothers recover from the temporary depression in one to seven days with no long-term consequences.

Rarer are the women who experience incapacitating symptoms, refusing to eat or to take care of their babies. Some have even tried to harm their newborns. Experts confirm that the women who have the more severe symptoms usually have a history of depressive episodes.

Elderly

In addition to abuse victims and women, people over the age of sixty suffer a higher rate of depression. Research has found that depression in the elderly is four times more

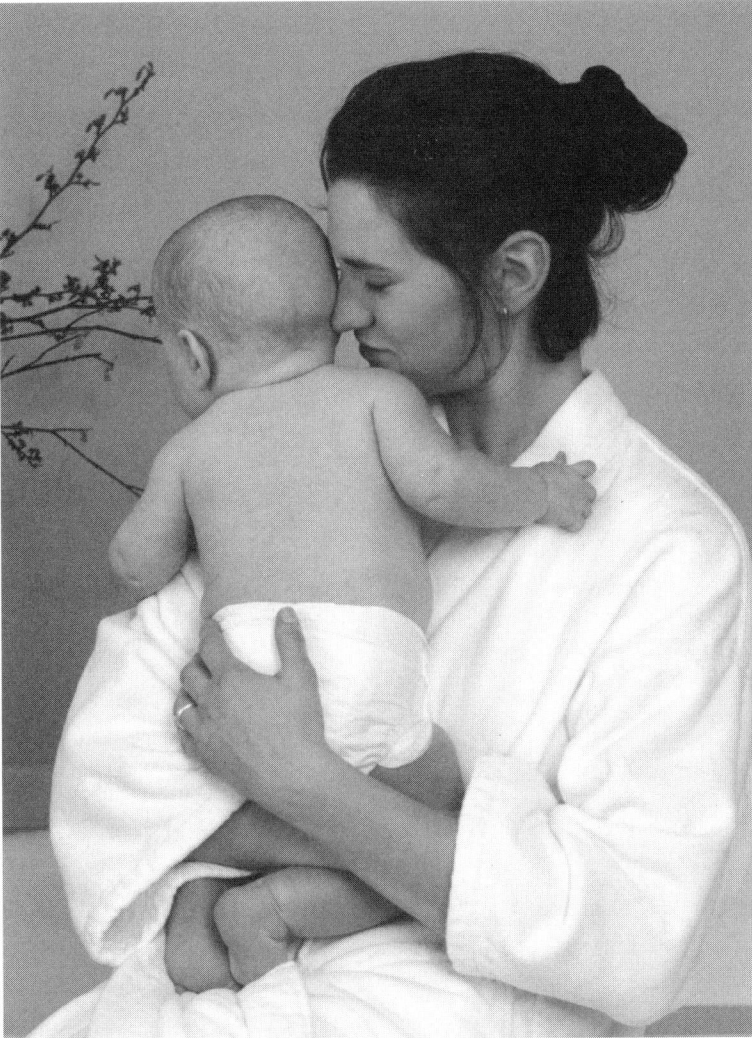

Changes in hormone levels during and after pregnancy may lead to mood swings and depression in women.

prevalent than in the general population. The period after age sixty is a time of great change when people may face retirement, deteriorating health, and the deaths of friends and siblings. These events may also bring about thoughts of their own mortality. These events, plus the hormonal changes that occur naturally with aging, make depression more common among the elderly.

In *Good News About Depression,* Dr. Gold states:

> Living into old age means contending with loss . . . of health, vigor, opportunities, strength, physical and mental prowess,

friends, spouses, siblings, work, earnings, independence, residences, and support networks. Loneliness, boredom, and helplessness threaten.[12]

Marguerite Parke, a ninety-year-old resident in a retirement village, wonders whether she has any business still living. "All my friends have died, my daughter has died, I can't work, I can't garden . . . what good am I?"[13]

A sense of loss and helplessness can cause such severe distress that many older people choose to take their own lives. Even though the elderly make up only 12 percent of the population, they constitute almost 25 percent of all suicides.

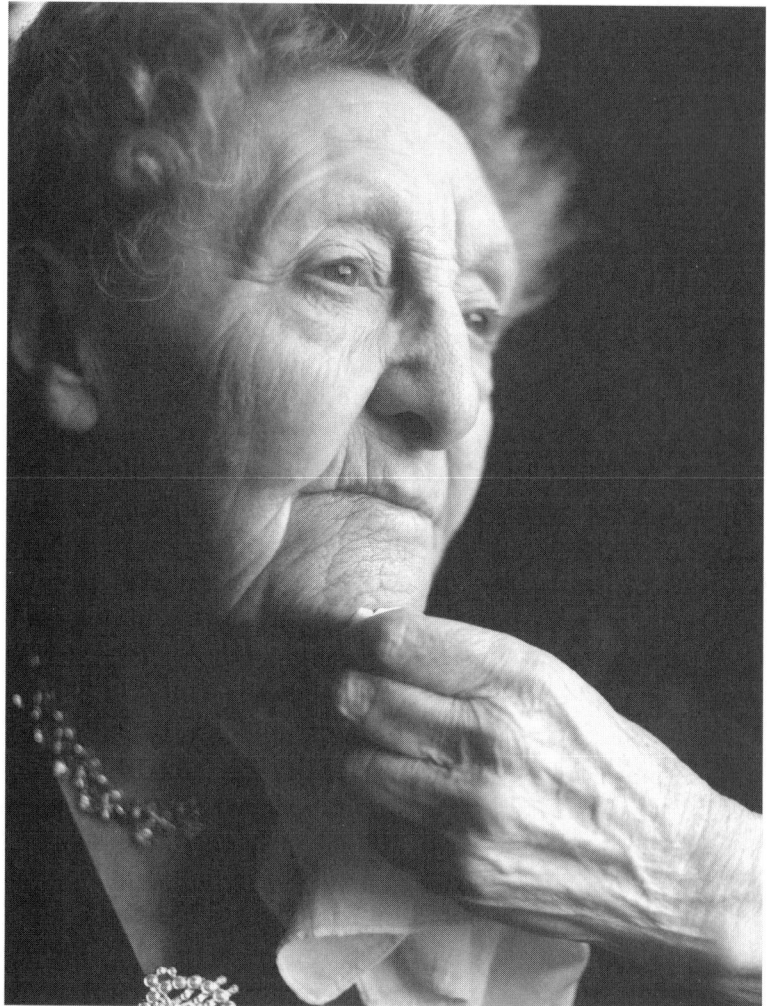

People over the age of sixty are four times more likely to suffer from depression, especially when they are physically weak or disabled.

High suicide rates among the elderly have been tied not only to profound life changes but also to changing serotonin levels. At least one study also indicates that the stresses of aging can depress even further the levels of this important neurotransmitter.

Using magnetic resonance imaging (MRI), a team of researchers from the University of Pittsburgh Medical Center made an interesting discovery. In people diagnosed with depression, they found an additional 55 percent decline in serotonin levels in several areas of the brain even after normal aging changes were taken into account. This led researchers to believe that stressful circumstances the elderly face contribute to reduced serotonin, which could account for the extreme hopeless feelings. In turn, the aggression often unleashed when serotonin is low may be reflected in the higher incidence of suicide, as despairing older people turn their violent impulses on themselves.

Children

Like the elderly, children also have a high potential for developing depression. While the experiences of older people and children differ markedly, these two groups share at least one source of frustration: the inability to control certain major events in life. The extreme stress associated with these events and the inability to control them put some children at high risk of developing depression.

Two decades ago, depression in children was largely unheard of. However, because of better research involving the biochemistry of depression, today psychiatrists believe more than three million American young people suffer some form of the disease. Unfortunately, symptoms are sometimes harder to detect in the young, and it often takes an attempted suicide to make parents and others aware of a young person's distress.

Symptoms in young people, which can include temper tantrums in toddlers and severe mood swings in teenagers, are often masked by cultural expectations. ("All babies fuss," friends will reassure a worried parent. "A moody fourteen-year-old—so what else is new?") Other symptoms

Young people are at risk for depression because they experience many events over which they have no control such as divorce, an unexpected family move, and deaths of family members.

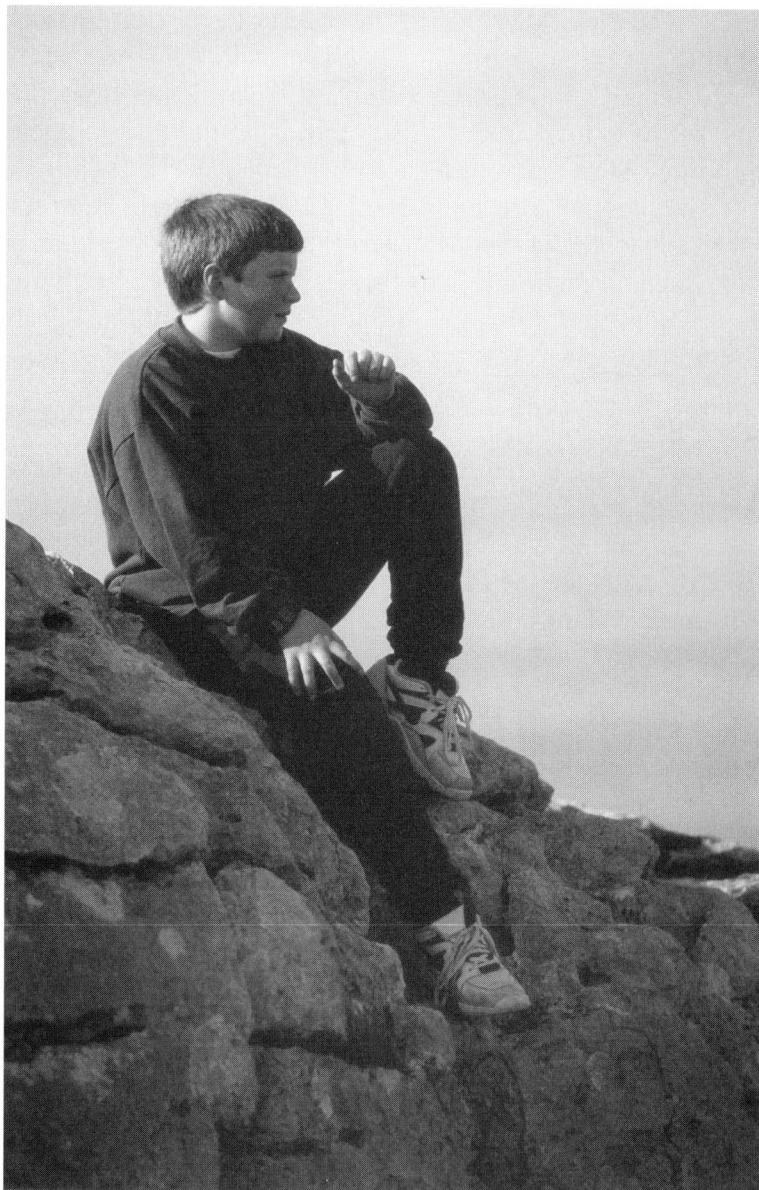

in children, including stomachaches and headaches, are similar to those of adults. Depression might show up in the sulky pout sessions in young children, or in the full-fledged rebellion of unhappy teenagers. Diagnosis is difficult because both the emotional and the physical clues reflect normal phases all young people go through.

Parents and other caregivers need to worry when episodes of misbehavior become consistent patterns. As with adults, young people who have a reduced ability to handle stress, and those who might have a genetic predisposition to depression, are potentially at risk for developing a depressive disorder.

One young girl, a daughter of a U.S. ambassador, exhibited wild mood swings and received many inaccurate diagnoses throughout her childhood before finally receiving treatment for bipolar disorder in her midteens. The stresses she had experienced (parental divorce, several relocations) are shared by many in her generation. But the biochemical makeup of the diplomat's daughter combined with the divorce and the frequent moves to cause severe mental anguish. This type of suffering can lead to other problems as children grow and try to hide their pain and negative feelings.

Many researchers today believe that the drug abuse among teenagers may be the result of years of untreated mood disorders. Virginia Hamilton, an addiction counselor connected with New York Hospital, says:

Source: National Alliance for Research on Schizophrenia and Depression, Myrna M. Weissman; Maurice Blackman, MB, FRCPC; *The Canadian Journal of CME.*

Facts About Mood Disorders in Children and Adolescents

▶ 7–14% of children will experience an episode of major depression before age 15

▶ 20–30% of adult bipolar patients report that their disorder began before the age of 20

▶ one-third of adolescents attending psychiatric clinics suffer from depression

▶ greater than 20% of adolescents in the general population suffer from emotional problems

▶ the onset of major depression is earlier in children of depressed parents (mean age of 12.7 years) compared with those of normal parents (mean age of 16.8 years)

A teenager suffering from depression may mask his or her feelings by drinking alcohol, taking drugs, or smoking cigarettes.

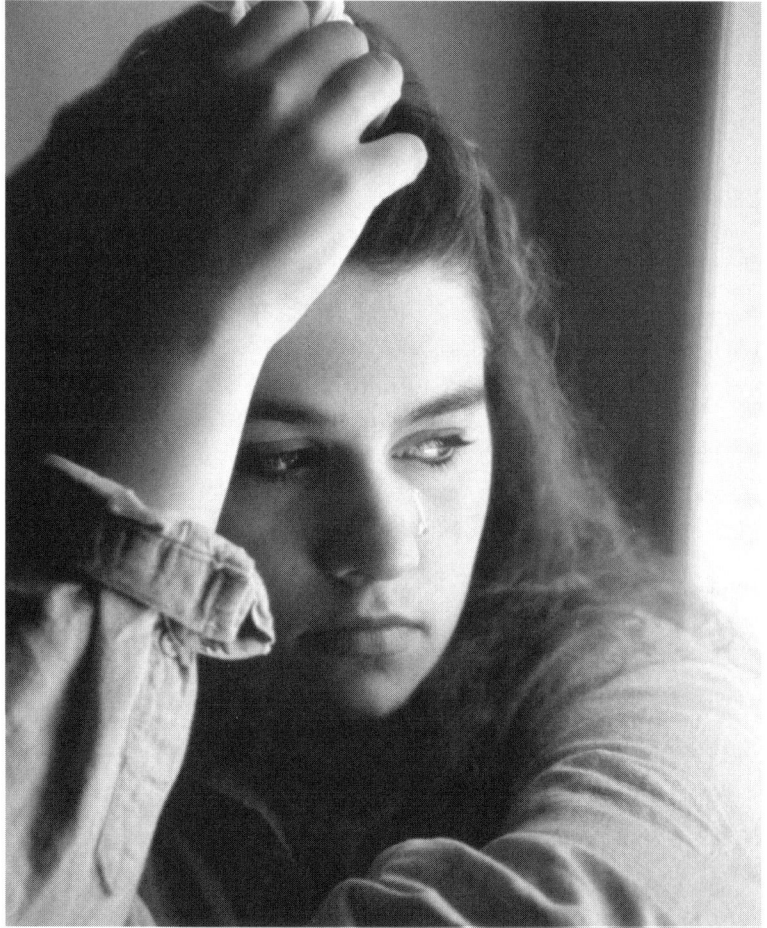

It has gotten complicated. These kids come in here on all kinds of street drugs. They have underlying psychiatric disorders that are very sophisticated—atypical [nontypical] depressions, bipolar disorders, atypical bipolar disorders.[14]

Reports like this lead some experts to believe that the addictions are not the major source of suffering. They suggest that depressive illnesses have caused some kids to find their own treatment in mind-numbing substances such as alcohol and other drugs. Some experts even believe teenagers who are depressed are more likely to begin smoking than teenagers who are not depressed.

Depression, which often begins at an early age, affects family relationships, school friendships, and often academic performance. When children do poorly in school, they may be placed at a lower learning level, which not only further hampers their self-esteem but, even worse, permits their depression to remain undiagnosed.

Greater awareness of all the high-risk groups may lead to more opportunities for treatment and reduce the number of people who live their lives under a cloud of undiagnosed depression.

4

Treating Depression

TREATMENT FOR DEPRESSION is often a trial-and-error process. Varying causes, symptoms, and body chemistries make it impossible for there to be a single treatment for everyone. The most common treatments today consist of medication, therapy, or some combination of both.

With accurate diagnosis and the right treatment, depression can be controlled. According to the American Psychiatric Association, approximately 85 percent of depression sufferers find relief with proper treatment. This represents a vast improvement over the medical field's ability to deal with depression from a decade ago, when treatment often failed or side effects hampered a patient's improvement. As one knowledgeable physician says:

> . . . we have managed to drastically reduce the long wait for therapeutic effectiveness; increase the odds against first time failure; prevent relapse for a vast number of patients; limit distressing side effects; and contribute to the storehouse of knowledge that can be applied to all depressed patients.[15]

However, getting people to enter the evaluation process can be an ordeal. Because people with depression often believe that their problems are due to weak will or to a personality flaw, they may not seek help at all.

Eleanor was a forty-year-old woman who struggled with feelings of sadness for over twenty-five years. She tried everything from meditation to cutting out coffee and eating only vegetables and fruits. She never considered going to a doctor, however, because she assumed her long-running sadness stemmed from her lifestyle or personality. Eleanor felt miserable; her body ached and she felt tired all the time. Finally, after a car accident, her depression became unmanageable, and she consulted a psychiatrist. He tried several medications before finally discovering a combination that eased Eleanor's depression: "I feel as if I've been ripped off my entire life because I was depressed for so long," she reports. "Now I have my sense of humor back. I feel great. I feel *normal*." [16]

The general public is not the only segment of society that is misinformed about depression. Some mental health professionals have not kept up with the latest research and are unaware of new ideas about causes, symptoms, and treatments for depression. Their failure to stay current with progress in the field can present problems for patients seeking help.

One woman, whose husband had committed suicide while in the grip of bipolar disorder, was no stranger to the signs

Men are less likely to seek treatment for symptoms of depression than are women. Today, depression is often treated with a combination of medications.

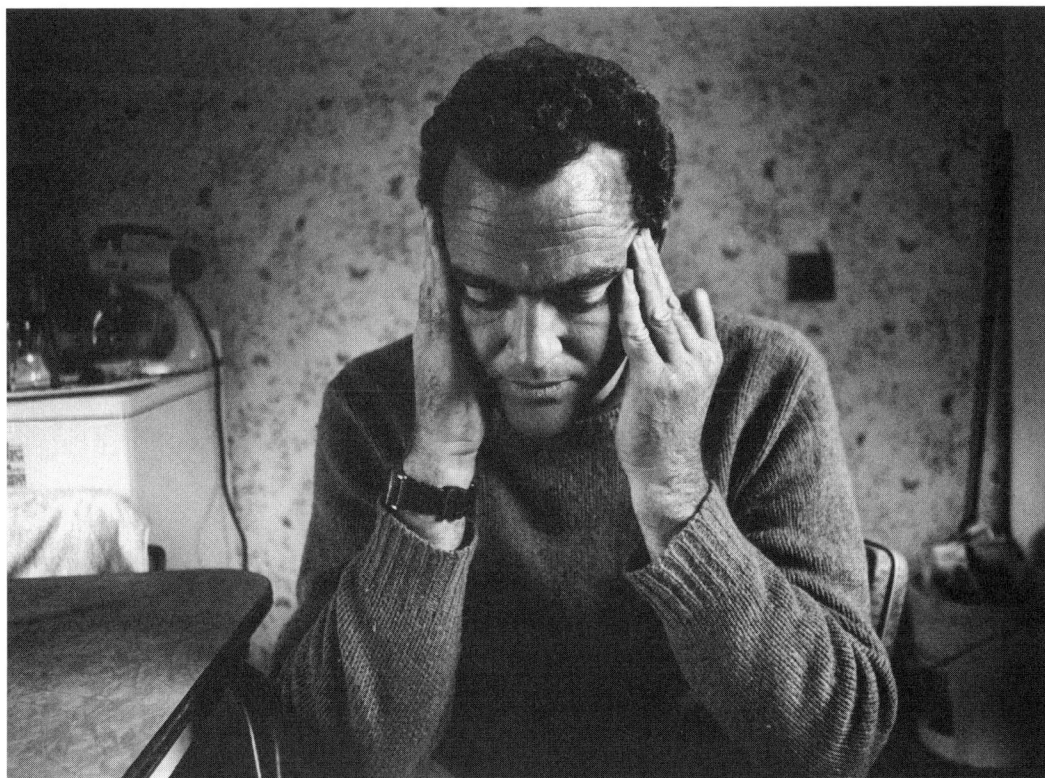

of depression. So, in the early 1990s, when her college-age daughter showed signs of depression, such as having difficulty getting out of bed to study, she took the girl to a psychiatrist. The psychiatrist determined that there was nothing wrong, other than normal exam apprehension. The woman chose another psychiatrist. The second doctor stated that the daughter had a less severe form of bipolar disorder than the type that had troubled her father and prescribed treatment. Soon the student became enthusiastic once more about her studies and about her life in general.

There is no one-size-fits-all approach to treating depression. Each patient is different and each requires a treatment plan tailored to his or her needs. Whatever the specifics of an individual treatment plan, most successful plans address the needs of mind and body and involve the patient in the decision-making process. As family therapist Kathryn Foster states:

> There's no question any longer that body and mind are interwoven. Healing depression takes time. Some people respond well to antidepressants. Others prefer to try psychotherapy. Occasionally, I might recommend both, along with an antidepressant so the patient can feel well enough to begin psychotherapy. Most important, they need to know the benefits of the medications and the different types of psychotherapy available.[17]

Drug treatment

One of the most common types of treatment for major depression is pharmacotherapy, which is the use of antidepressants or other drugs. Drug treatment for depression goes back to at least the late 1800s, when the drug of choice for "manic depression" was lithium. Lithium helped to even out the extreme high and low moods of manic depressives, as victims of bipolar disorder were then called; but it worked in only about half the patients who used it, and it had many unpleasant side effects. Nausea, hand trembling, and muscle weakness were common, especially in the early weeks of treatment. One of the most disturbing side effects was memory loss. About one-third of the people who take lithium experience some memory loss, reports Dr. Charles L. Bowden, a psychiatrist at the University of Texas Health Science Center in San Antonio.

Antidepressants

In recent years, antidepressants have replaced lithium as the most common drug for treatment of major depression. These drugs are designed to maintain a proper balance of serotonin in the brain and to reduce the symptoms of depression. Antidepressants are not addictive or habit forming. Thus when used as directed, they are a safe method of treatment, even for people who need to use them for many years.

People who take antidepressants experience various levels of relief and additional effects (so-called side effects), as well. This is why patients often have to try several different drugs and dosages before finding the best combination.

The people who have the biggest problem with side effects are those who have to take antidepressants for long periods of time. Some who experienced uncomfortable weight gain or skin rash may abandon the therapy because of a low tolerance for these effects. However, most people are willing to put up with minor physical discomforts in favor of the benefits of the medication.

Most treatment-related effects, such as restlessness or dizziness, go away over time. Some can be lessened with a simple reduction in dosage. Sometimes changing the time of day a medicine is taken, or dividing doses into smaller portions to be taken more often throughout the day, will eliminate unwanted reactions.

Melissa Kluth, who suffered with depression for years before starting on antidepressants, is thankful that she can safely take her medication for as long as she needs it. She says her behavior gets out of control when she has tried to go without the antidepressant:

> When I'm off the medication, if you say anything to me, I get angry. I scream and yell and kick and throw chairs. When I'm on the medication, I'm fine; nothing bothers me.[18]

As helpful as the new medications are for the treatment of depression, most mental health professionals urge doctors who prescribe such drugs to advise their patients to seek some form of counseling, as well.

How Antidepressants Work

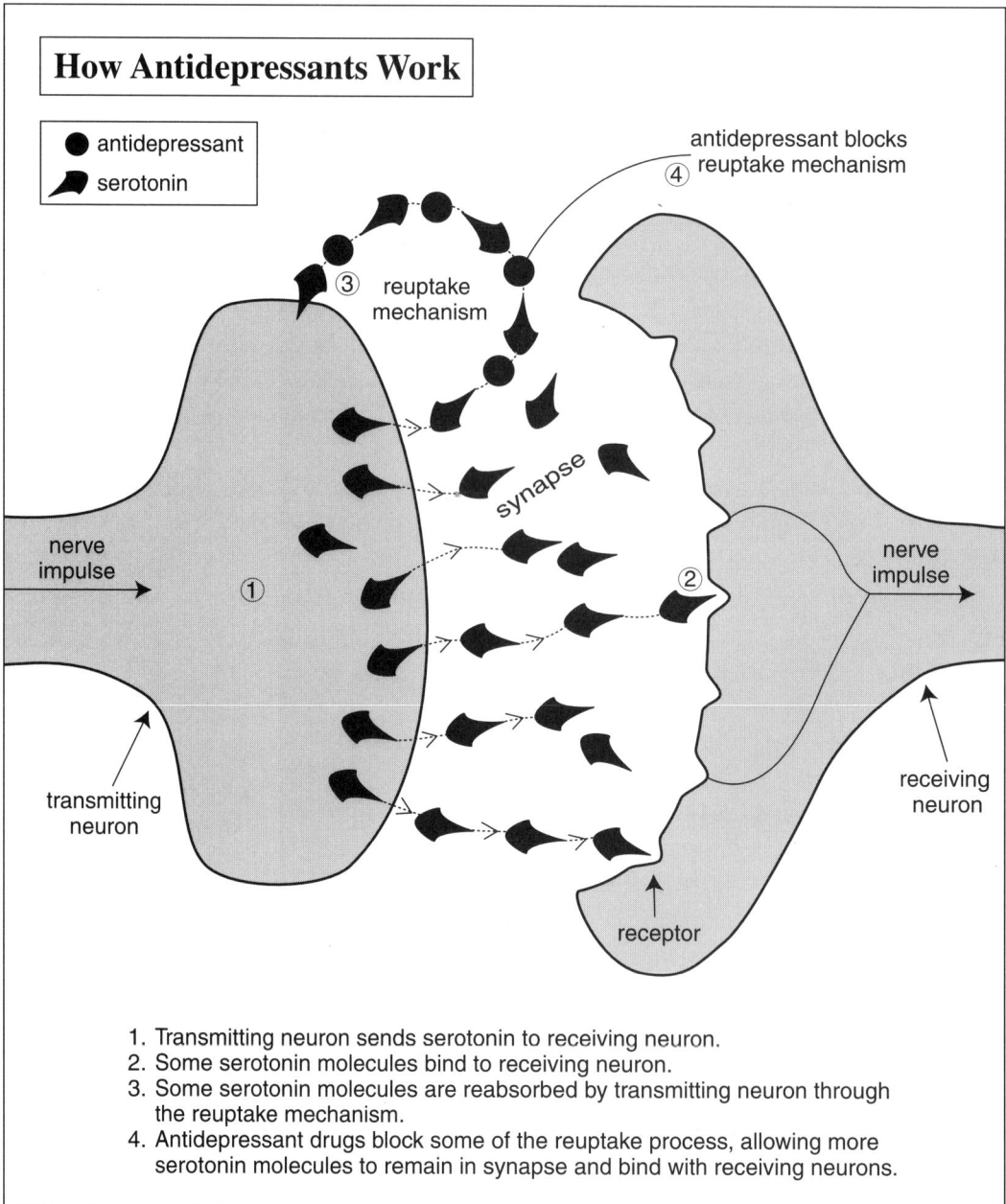

1. Transmitting neuron sends serotonin to receiving neuron.
2. Some serotonin molecules bind to receiving neuron.
3. Some serotonin molecules are reabsorbed by transmitting neuron through the reuptake mechanism.
4. Antidepressant drugs block some of the reuptake process, allowing more serotonin molecules to remain in synapse and bind with receiving neurons.

Psychotherapy

Psychotherapy uses the so-called talking therapies to help depression sufferers change maladaptive thinking patterns. With research pointing out the brain's tendency to stay locked in a given thinking pattern, even a negative one, many mental health experts believe that psychotherapy can help depression sufferers learn positive patterns of thinking, behaving, and communicating.

Three primary types of therapy are used to bring about such changes: cognitive, behavioral, and interpersonal. In the most common form, cognitive therapy, a therapist helps the client to work toward a shift in thinking.

Therapists using cognitive therapy help people learn ways to focus on positive thoughts, rather than relying on their habitual negative thinking patterns. First, the therapist helps the client identify his or her negative thoughts, which often are revealed in untrue generalizations such as "I can never do anything right." These comments often come from well-respected, successful people who nevertheless think that any small mistake or inadequacy erases their right to exist.

As the next step, the therapist helps the person change the "automatic" negative thought patterns. Therapists often encourage depressed clients to keep a log of their thoughts and feelings, and to try to spot patterns in the types of event that cause their low moods. They bring those insights to the therapist and together the two work on ways to block out or replace automatic negative thinking with more positive, realistic thinking.

For example, one depressed man realized that his low moods stemmed from situations in which he felt that he had not performed well enough. His therapist encouraged him to write down on an index card all the things he did well, and to keep that card in his wallet. Later, when any negative thoughts crept in, he whipped out the card and "replaced" the characterizations of personal inadequacy with his own positive traits from the card.

Practicing strategies like this can help depressed people to overcome their low moods, sometimes without medications.

A therapist works with a depressed patient. Therapists may try a number of techniques, including behavioral or cognitive therapy, to help a depressed person.

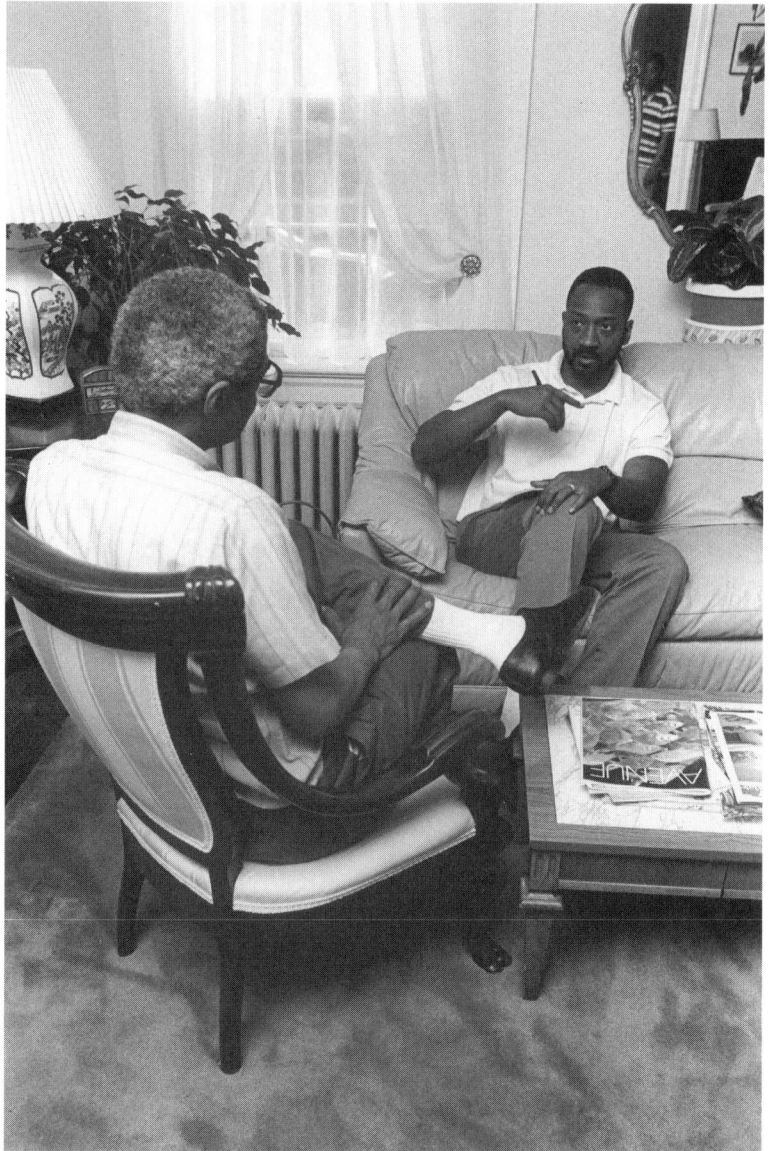

Second in popularity to cognitive therapy, behavioral therapy focuses on what people do and why. When any faulty behavior patterns are recognized and monitored, certain coping strategies can be used to ease the negative behaviors and the negative thinking behind them that cause depression. John Kelsoe, assistant professor of psychiatry at the University of California, San Diego, says:

Every thought we think alters the biology of our brain. Every mood we have must represent some kind of chemical difference in our brain. So, behavior and brain changes mirror each other very closely. Under some circumstances, you can measure the changes in the brain chemistry that result from a change in thought or attitude or action.[19]

Using behavioral therapy, therapists might encourage depressed clients to identify their low moods by the undesirable behavior that tends to accompany them. Some people overeat. Some withdraw from friends or relatives. Some abuse alcohol or drugs. After composing these lists of behaviors, clients discuss with their therapists the thoughts that triggered the self-destructive actions. This process allows them to work out ways to "switch" from a negative behavior to a positive behavior.

A frazzled secretary who used to seek relief in the chocolate bars stocked in the company's snack machine has found another way to deal with stress. She still digs in her purse for quarters, but now takes a quick "time out" walk down the hall. When she returns, she deposits the quarters in a see-through bank on her desk, to save the money for something special. Now when she takes a break from stress, instead of consuming hundreds of extra calories and fleeing from the negative situation, she returns to the scene, pleased to be able to do something positive for herself with the money she would have spent on chocolate.

While cognitive and behavior therapies concentrate on either thinking patterns or behavioral patterns, the third therapeutic mode combines the two. Interpersonal therapy also centers on the depressed person's relationships with others and tries to help the client improve communication and relational skills.

A depressed woman binges on snacks while remaining in bed. A depressed person may turn to food to alleviate emotional pain.

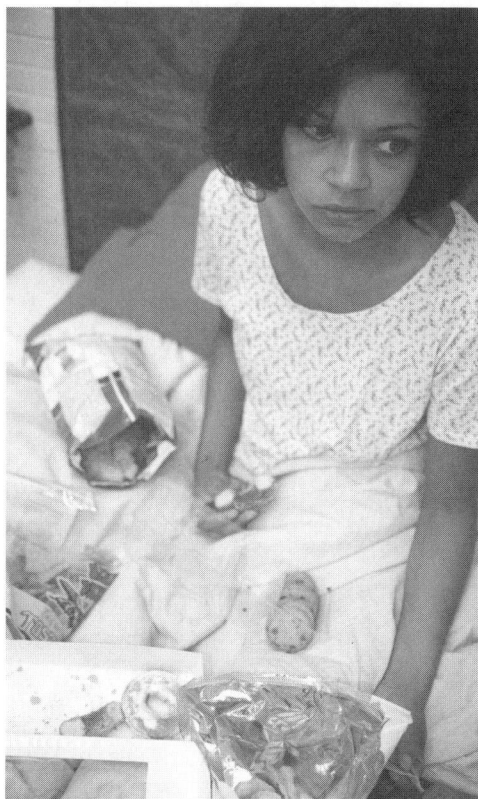

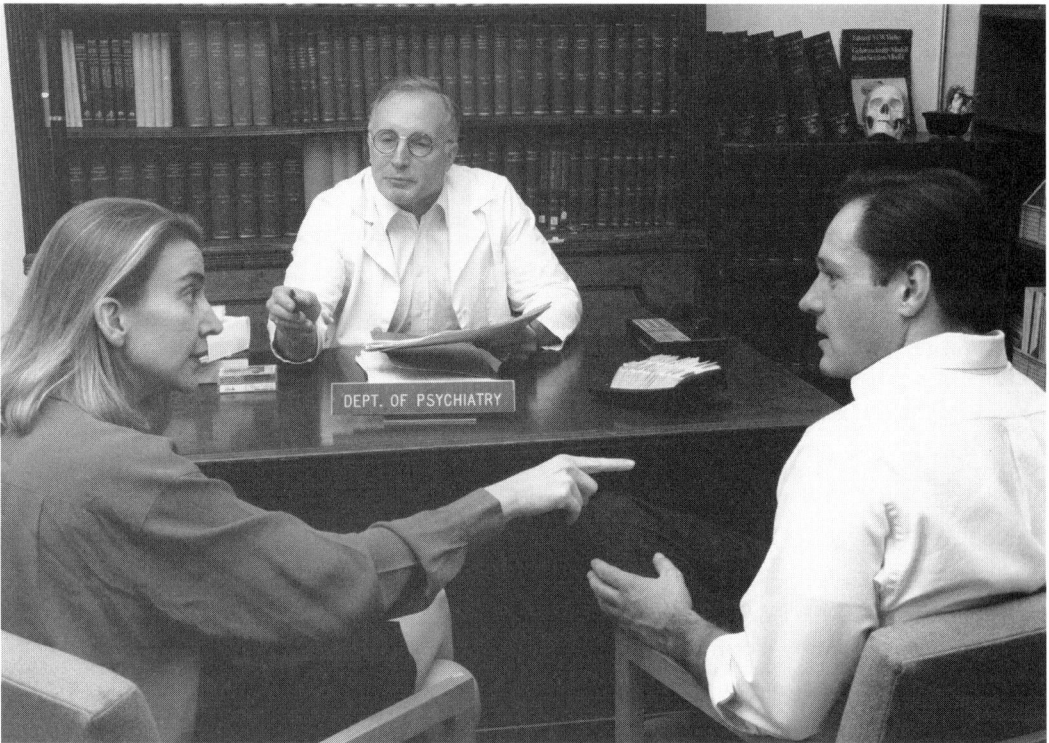

A couple tries to solve their marital problems by speaking to a therapist. Such therapy is called interpersonal therapy.

A therapist will use interpersonal therapy to emphasize specific issues bothering a person in a current situation. Then the therapist will teach behaviors intended to enhance existing relationships. Often people whose depression comes from feeling that their lives are out of their control respond well to this type of therapy. Interpersonal therapy is particularly effective for people who are grieving the loss of loved ones. It also works well for newlyweds or new parents, or middle-aged people forced to become caregivers to an elderly parent or a disabled spouse. Sometimes conflicts in work or personal relationships are also helped with interpersonal therapy.

One woman's mild depression stemmed from a sense of not having control over her work environment. She felt trapped into listening to coworkers complain and realized that she had allowed herself to be the silent listener. After a few sessions of therapy, she was able to devise a couple of compassionate phrases to offer when cornered by complainers. She would say these phrases and then add, "Hope things work out better for you," or "I'll be praying for you," to ease herself out of time-consuming, emotionally draining conversations.

The positive results of treatment for depression can often come from one or any combination of therapies. The important element is that changes occur because the therapies prove effective in altering the thought patterns typical of depression. When those thoughts change, the neurotransmitters return to normal levels, and the person being treated has a better chance for living a happier life.

5

Alternative
Treatments

ALTHOUGH THE MOST common treatment therapies have a high success rate, not everyone responds to them. When the most frequently prescribed medication or therapy fails to bring relief, many depressed people look for alternatives. Some of these approaches have been the subject of scientific study and have shown good results. Others have not been through controlled tests, but anecdotal evidence suggest benefits. Today, many alternative therapies for treating depression have gained acceptance, and studies continue in an effort to determine the effectiveness of others.

Electroconvulsive therapy

The most common treatment for severe depression in the 1930s and 1940s was electroconvulsive therapy, ECT, or electroshock therapy. ECT is still used today, but it is no longer considered a standard treatment.

In ECT, electrodes, which are small conductors of electricity, are connected to specific points on a person's scalp. The leads, or wires attached to the actual conducting units, are attached at the other end to a machine that distributes electricity into the brain. The electrical current is transmitted in a series of pulses, each lasting about two seconds and causing brief convulsions, or muscle contractions.

Experts think the sudden application of electricity destroys the electrical patterns of the brain. They believe the

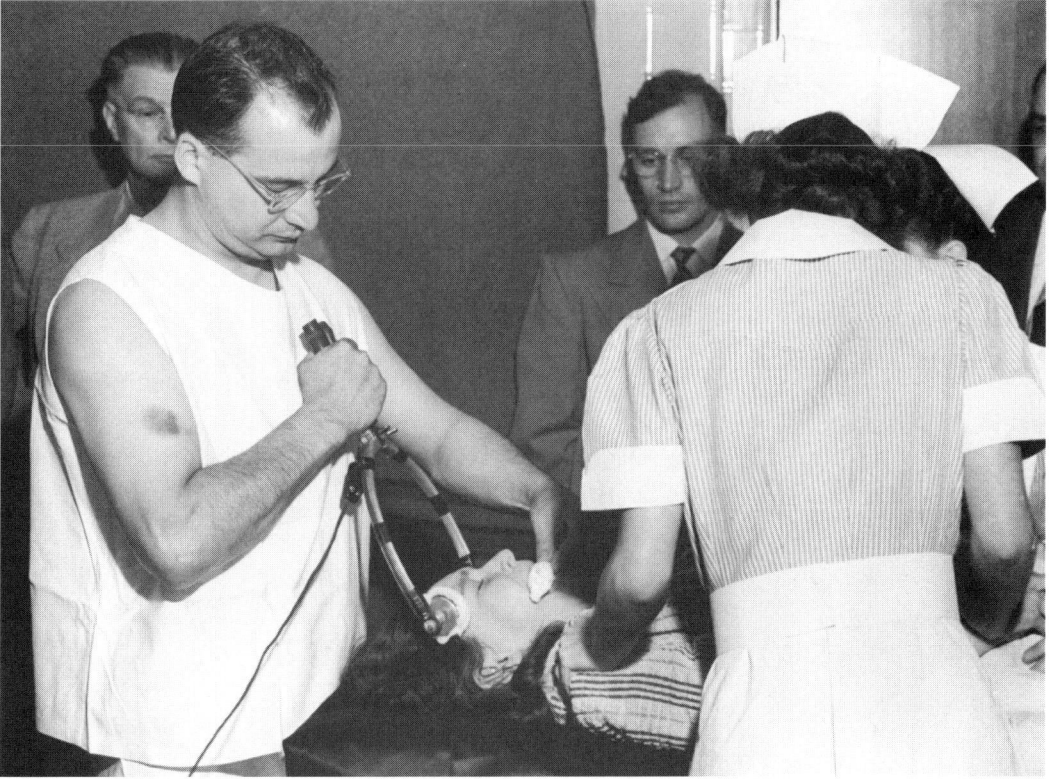

electricity exerts an effect similar to that of the antidepressants. Although ECT was successful in the past in calming patients and evening out their high and low moods, the treatment as originally administered was severe.

When ECT was introduced, many patients lost teeth or fractured their vertebrae during the intense convulsions brought on by unnecessarily high electrical charges. Some people were more traumatized by the treatment than helped by it.

Ted Chabasinski, now a lawyer in his sixties, was given shock treatments at New York's Bellevue Hospital when he was only six years old, living in a foster home. Young Ted had shown signs of being withdrawn, and because his mother suffered from mental illness, doctors decided the boy had to have a similar condition. ECT was performed on him based on that inadequate evaluation. Chabasinski recalls:

A doctor treats a depressed patient with electroconvulsive therapy (ECT) in 1949. ECT was once standard treatment for depression but is now used in modified form for those who do not respond to newer therapies.

It made me want to die. I remember they would stick a rag in my mouth so I wouldn't bite through my tongue and that it took three attendants to hold me down.[20]

Revelations of traumatized patients and the development of antidepressants weakened the appeal of ECT. Today, ECT is viewed as an effective alternative for patients who have not had success with the newer, standard treatments. Numerous studies list improvement in 70 to 80 percent of patients who choose the procedure, which is given in a more humane fashion and after more thorough evaluation than in the past. Today, patients are not conscious when they receive the treatment; they are given general anesthesia, and also muscle relaxants, to help offset the headaches that often follow ECT. Also, with the help of advanced technology, modern ECT machines can better regulate the electrical impulses that enter the brain, and monitor brain function, while the treatment is being performed. These procedures help control the flow of electricity, to ensure that a patient does not accidentally get too much.

Modern ECT techniques are safer and more effective than methods used in the past.

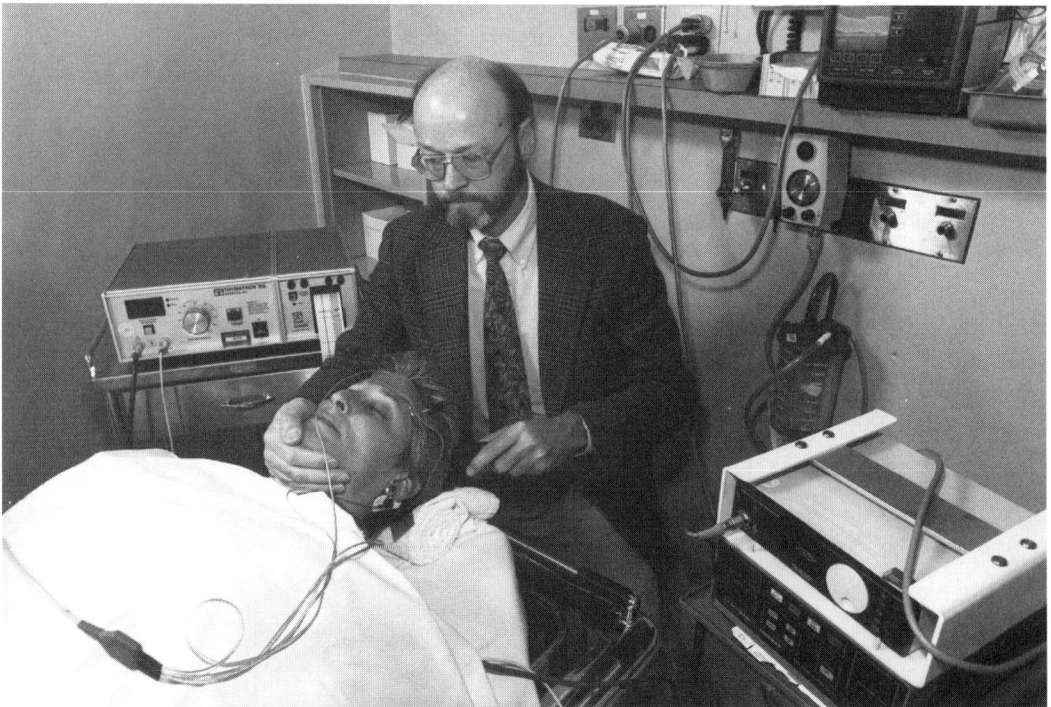

However, even with better ECT equipment, one problem remains: the possibility of memory loss after treatment. Some people have difficulty remembering events that happened a few months before or after receiving this therapy. Others have trouble remembering even significant events in their past. One woman couldn't recall the funeral of her two-year-old son, who had drowned in a backyard swimming pool.

And yet, others experience no memory loss. Experts disagree about the effect of ECT on memory. Since people who have severe depression also suffer problems with their overall thinking processes, it is hard to be certain whether the memory loss is due to ECT treatments or is simply another symptom of the disease. Even so, ECT relieves many people of severe or chronic depression.

Advocating ECT

Jennie Forehand, a delegate to the Maryland state legislature, is a strong believer in the usefulness of ECT. Shortly after Forehand's father died, her now widowed mother began to withdraw from her circle of family and friends. The older woman's behavior became erratic, and before long symptoms of depression were evident. Forehand spent months taking her mother to doctors, but several antidepressant treatments proved to be unsuccessful.

Finally, at the suggestion of a colleague, Forehand took her mother to Maryland's premier medical institution, the hospital associated with the medical school of Johns Hopkins University. By this time, Forehand had asked the people who were caring for her mother to maintain a daily record of diet and behavior.

The researchers at Hopkins used that diary, plus a six-page letter Forehand had written about her mother's history, to determine that ECT offered the best hope for relief. Forehand's mother had seven shock treatments in all and memory loss was not a problem. Forehand says:

> It was absolutely wonderful. So many people are afraid of shock treatment, but it's so different and so much better than it used to be. . . .

> A lot of people talk of that [memory loss] as being one of the drawbacks. But she remembers everything: past, present, everything. I have not seen any downside. . . . I think that electric shock used to be considered a medieval thing, just a terrible thing to do to people. And they did it in state institutions, almost as a punishment. But I am a terrific advocate for ECT because I saw the good that came from it.[21]

Many mental health professionals agree with Forehand's assessment of ECT. Despite its history, and its association with memory loss, ECT is an effective treatment for prompt relief of severe depression; people who have made dangerous suicide attempts or are experiencing psychotic delusions or hallucinations also can benefit. Although the number of those who suffer these harrowing depressive episodes is small, in such extreme cases, ECT still ranks high in selection and success.

Phototherapy

While advanced technology and a greater understanding of depression have given new life to ECT, health professionals and patients are also exploring the use of new therapies. Phototherapy is one relatively new alternative treatment, in which sunlight, or bright artificial light, is used to help alleviate symptoms of seasonal depression. This type of depression is a mild, low-level disorder that affects people during the fall and winter months. It is commonly referred to as seasonal affective disorder (SAD), and people so diagnosed report extreme tiredness, loneliness, and sadness.

SAD was researched in the mid-1970s by Dr. Norman E. Rosenthal and categorized as a mild depression in the early 1980s. Rosenthal, a physician, believes people are affected by their environment, noting that just as hibernating animals change their behavior during the winter months, some people react to the lengthening and shortening of days by expressing a different set of behaviors. In his book, *Winter Blues,* he states:

> In their infinite variety of nature, people, like other creatures, are all different. Some show little change with the revolving year, while others react to seasonal changes with exquisite

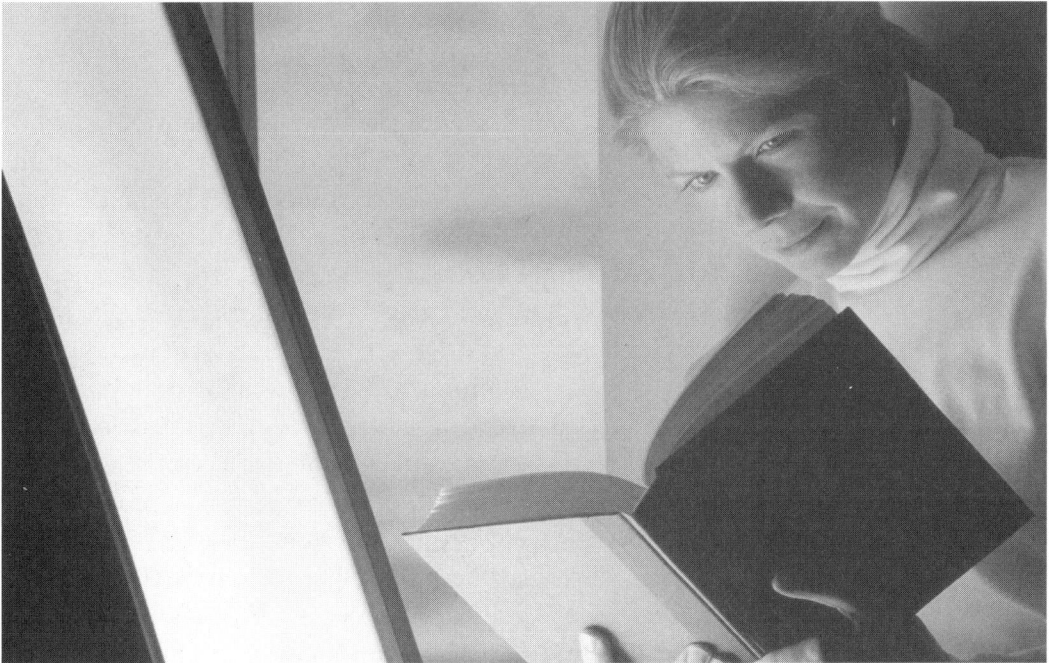

A woman reads near a box that gives off a bright, artificial light. People who suffer from SAD, a temporary depression that occurs during the fall and winter months, can relieve their symptoms with the help of light therapy.

sensitivity. There is no shortage of examples in the plant and animal world of creatures reacting to changes in light, heat, or moisture. People who experience marked seasonal changes have no reason to feel alone. Even among our fellow humans there are millions with such strong reactions. My colleagues and I have estimated that perhaps as many as 20 percent of the U.S. population—thirty-six million people—experience some diminished function or impaired quality of life in response to winter. [22]

During the early 1990s, hundreds of thousands of people in North America participated in a medical survey that included questions about their moods during the fall and winter months. Nearly 20 percent listed symptoms consistent with SAD. Most of these people lived in the northern areas, where the number of sunny daytime hours is markedly low in the fall and winter months.

Further research showed that higher levels of light affected respiration, blood pressure, body temperature, and most importantly, the production of melatonin, a hormone released from a gland in the brain. High levels of light in the early morning regulate melatonin production later at night when it is dark. Since low melatonin levels can cause depression, phototherapy has been found helpful in relieving many SAD sufferers.

The most common phototherapy treatment consists of exposure to light similar to outdoor brightness for 30 minutes every morning, before 10 o'clock. This can be done either by taking a brief walk or by sitting within two and a half feet of a light box made especially for this purpose. Other devices, known as dawn simulators, are night lights fitted with timers and dimmers. The units turn on automatically at 4 A.M. and emit a soft glow—an artificial dawn—which brightens over the next two to three hours. In one very small study, some subjects who used phototherapy reported significant relief after two weeks.

Phototherapy has proven to be beneficial to SAD sufferers and is currently being used in research for possible treatment of nonseasonal disorders. Although these studies are incomplete, researchers are hopeful phototherapy will aid other depression sufferers.

Vitamins

Relief from depression has also come from alternative remedies, such as vitamins and herbal therapies. The most well documented of the vitamin therapies is the use of B vitamins.

Research has confirmed that B vitamins are crucial to proper brain function and that deficiencies can cause symptoms of depression. Correcting inadequate levels in the body can help fend off depression and maintain a long-term resistance to recurring episodes. Zoltan P. Rona, a physician who is an expert in alternative medicines, states in a recent article:

Depression can often be healed naturally. A number of recent studies have reported that there is a definite benefit to be gained by giving vitamin B_{12} to patients suffering from depression, fatigue and mental illnesses of other kinds.[23]

Some people have found that taking vitamins, especially B vitamins, can help fend off feelings of depression.

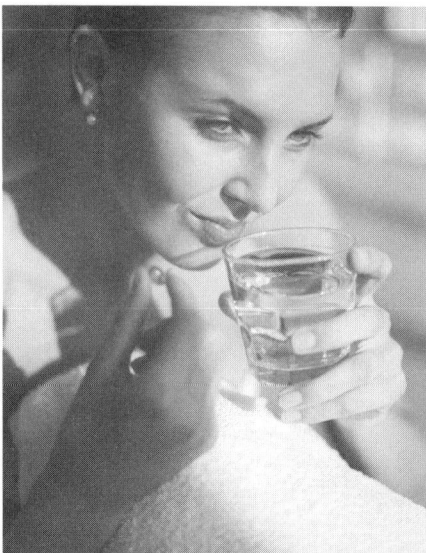

Rona also points out that B_{12} is not the only natural therapy that is useful in treating depression. The body also needs adequate levels of the other B complex vitamins, vitamin C, biotin, folic acid, calcium, copper, iron, magnesium, and potassium to ward off symptoms of depression. Deficiencies in any of these substances can alter the levels of chemicals in the body, which in turn could cause the brain's serotonin levels to drop and bring on symptoms of depression.

Herbal therapies

Another natural therapy for depression is *Hypericum perforatum,* the herbal remedy known as St. John's wort (root). Recently German scientists discovered that this plant, which has been used for centuries as an aid for healing wounds, also appears to regulate serotonin levels, much like a synthetic antidepressant. In Germany, doctors often prescribe St. John's wort for mild to moderate depression. St. John's wort is less well known in the United States, but researchers have begun studying its effectiveness as a treatment for depression.

A 1996 report published in the *British Medical Journal* listed results from a study conducted at the Audie Murphy Veterans Hospital in San Antonio, Texas. Out of the 1,751 participants, 55 percent of those who took St. John's wort experienced relief from their depression—a success rate similar to that of the synthetic antidepressants. The major differences between the natural antidepressant and the prescription drugs are found in the side effects and the cost. Possible unwanted effects produced by St. John's wort are mild (minor stomachache and dry mouth) compared to those due to prescription medicines. And the cost of a month's treatment with *Hypericum* runs only about $10—much less than other medications.

Ginkgo is another herbal remedy thought to have some effect on symptoms of depression. The active ingredient is extracted from ginkgo trees *(Ginkgo biloba),* which are found in China. Although there have not been many controlled studies with ginkgo, many alternative medicine specialists believe the herb normalizes the brain's serotonin levels. They base this assumption on the number of patients whose depression has been relieved after using ginkgo. However, more research is needed regarding St. John's wort and ginkgo before the benefits and potential additional effects can be compared to those of traditional treatments for depression.

Mood elevation

Perhaps the least researched and most skimpily documented therapies for depression are known as mood-elevating therapies. Mood elevation can be defined as creating or increasing a positive emotional attitude in a person who is feeling down as a result of the symptoms of depression. These psychological boosts help increase positive thought patterns. Some researchers believe these simple alterations will balance the biochemicals necessary to relieve depression. As with the herbal remedies, however, relatively few controlled studies have been published. This lack of a sizable body of research causes some doctors to bypass the mood-elevating therapies if another treatment option will work for a patient. But mood-elevating treatments have helped some people to conquer depression.

One of the oldest known practices of elevating mood is the use of meditation and relaxation. The techniques involve using pleasant imagery, such as visualizing peaceful surroundings, to help create a happier mood. "Many studies have shown mood elevation in depressed people who regularly elicit the relaxation response,"[24] says Dr. Herbert Benson, a Harvard researcher who did much to increase the acceptance of meditation in the American medical communities.

Another mood-elevating therapy features odors produced by the oils of certain plants. In this treatment, called aromatherapy, selected natural odors are released to create an atmosphere of pleasant sensual reactions. These reactions are thought to encourage positive thoughts, which then alter the brain chemicals. One study done in Japan reported very positive responses among 12 men hospitalized with serious depression, who were taking antidepressants and also exposed to strong citrus fragrance.

Therapeutic touch is a term given for massaging muscles to increase muscle relaxation. This muscle relaxation therapy creates a calmer perspective and positive attitude. At the Touch Research Institute at the Miami Medical School in Florida, women experiencing serious postpartum depression were given twenty-minute Swedish massages twice a week. The women soon found their moods improved, and researchers noted a corresponding decrease in the biochemical substances known informally as "stress hormones."

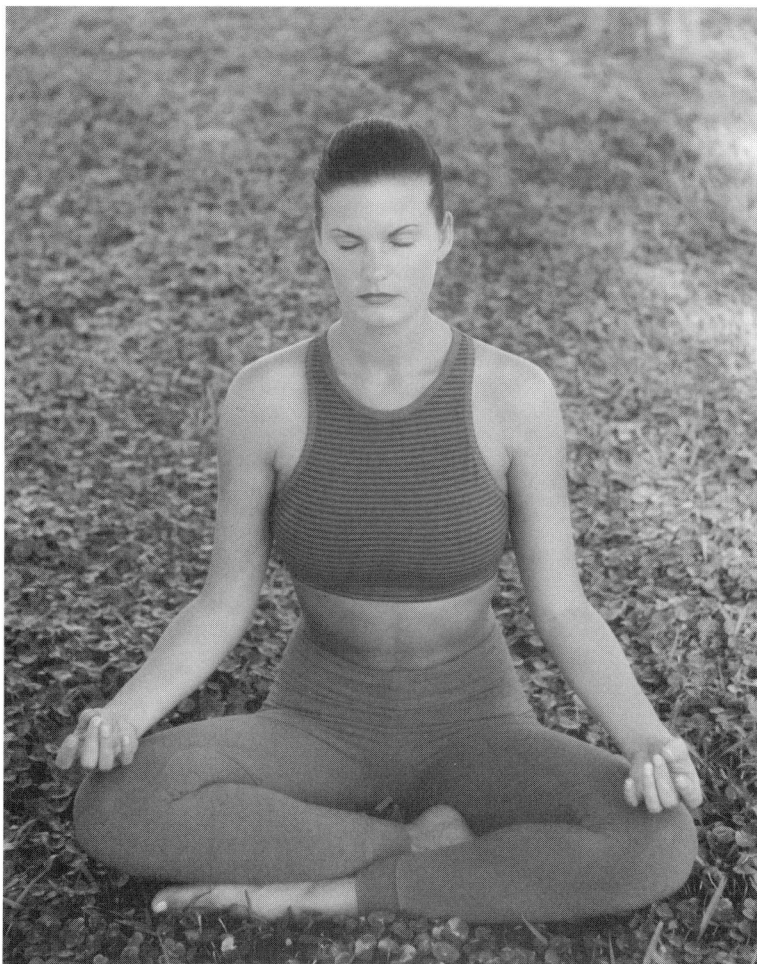

Meditation helps some depressed people relax and improve their mood.

Music is one of the oldest mood-elevating therapies. In biblical times, young David, a shepherd boy, was brought to King Saul to play his harp to help calm the king's bad moods. More recently, music therapy has been studied as a form of stress relief for older people suffering serious depression.

In one study, a group received weekly visits from music therapists who played music and taught other ways to manage stress. Another group was given taped music, followed up with weekly phone calls from music therapists who offered stress management tips. A third control group received stress management tips but no music therapy aids, and its members showed less improvement in mood than the two groups that were exposed to some form of music.

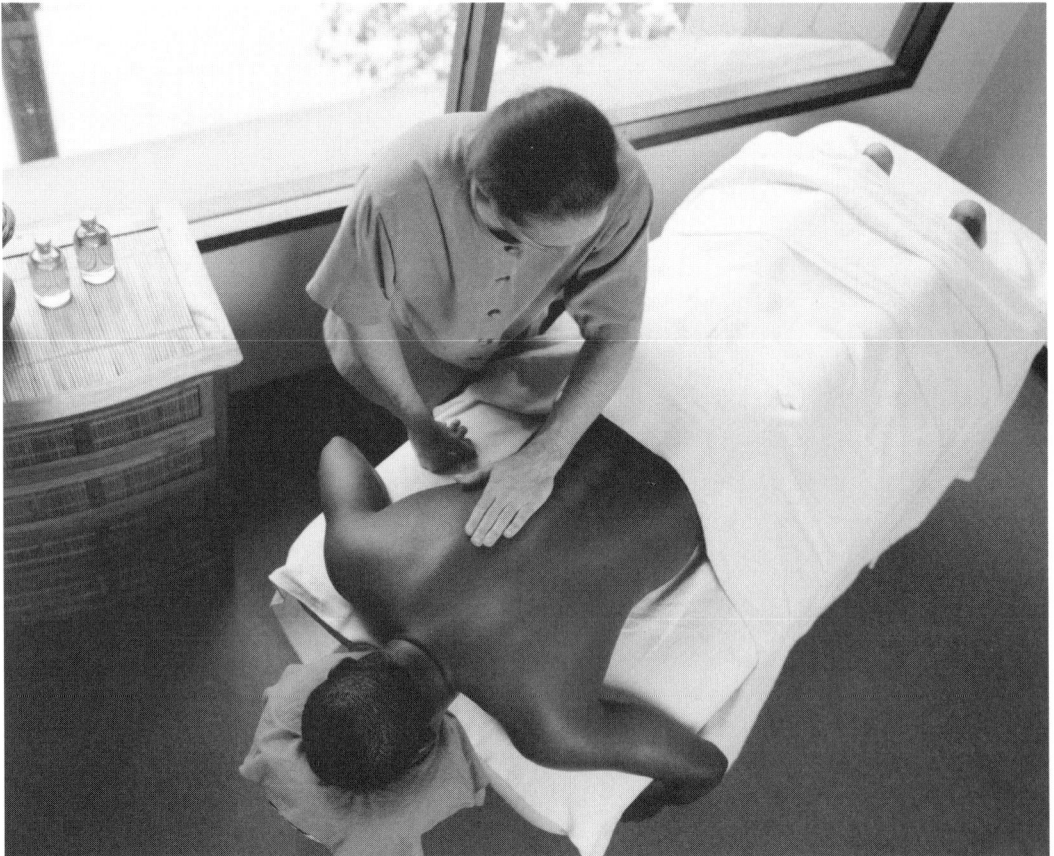

A massage therapist works with a patient. Therapeutic touch is one alternative therapy for depression.

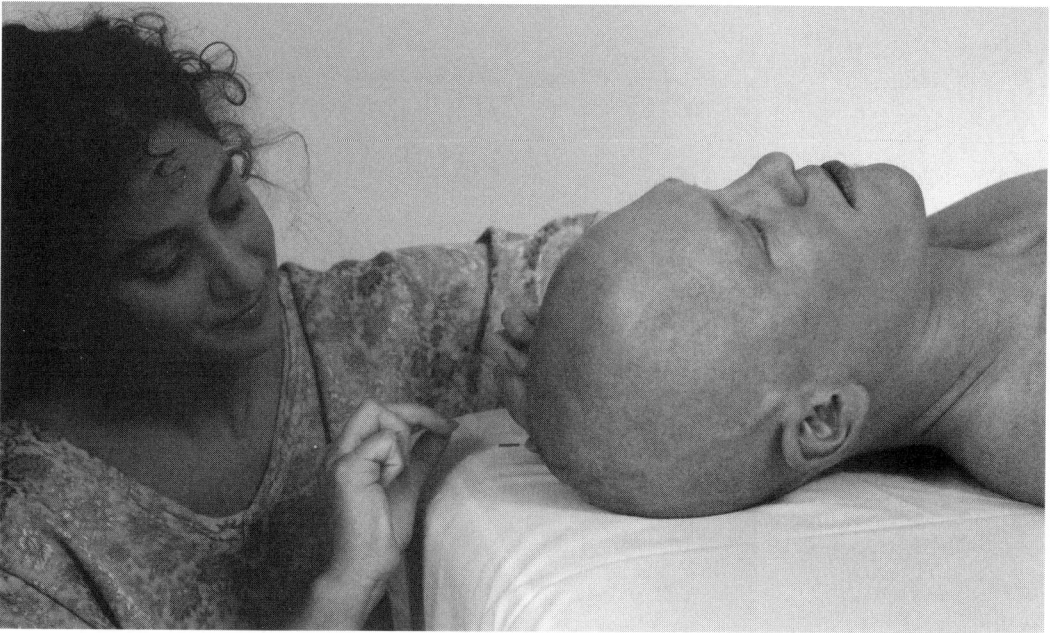

Acupuncture is the ancient Chinese art of inserting fine needles into specific points on the body. It is the only alternative therapy endorsed by the United Nations World Health Organization as a beneficial treatment for depression. Recently, at the University of Arizona, John Allen, an assistant professor of psychology, studied thirty-four women who had been diagnosed with major depression but were not being treated with antidepressants. The women were divided into three groups. One-third, the control group, did not receive any acupuncture. One-third received needle insertions, but not at points recommended for treating depression. The third group received acupuncture at the depression points, and these women showed significantly greater mood elevation than those in either of the other groups. This evidence and research from other studies earned acupuncture its high recommendation as an alternative treatment for depression.

Exercise

Although not normally classified as a therapy, exercise has received much attention for its effect on endorphins.

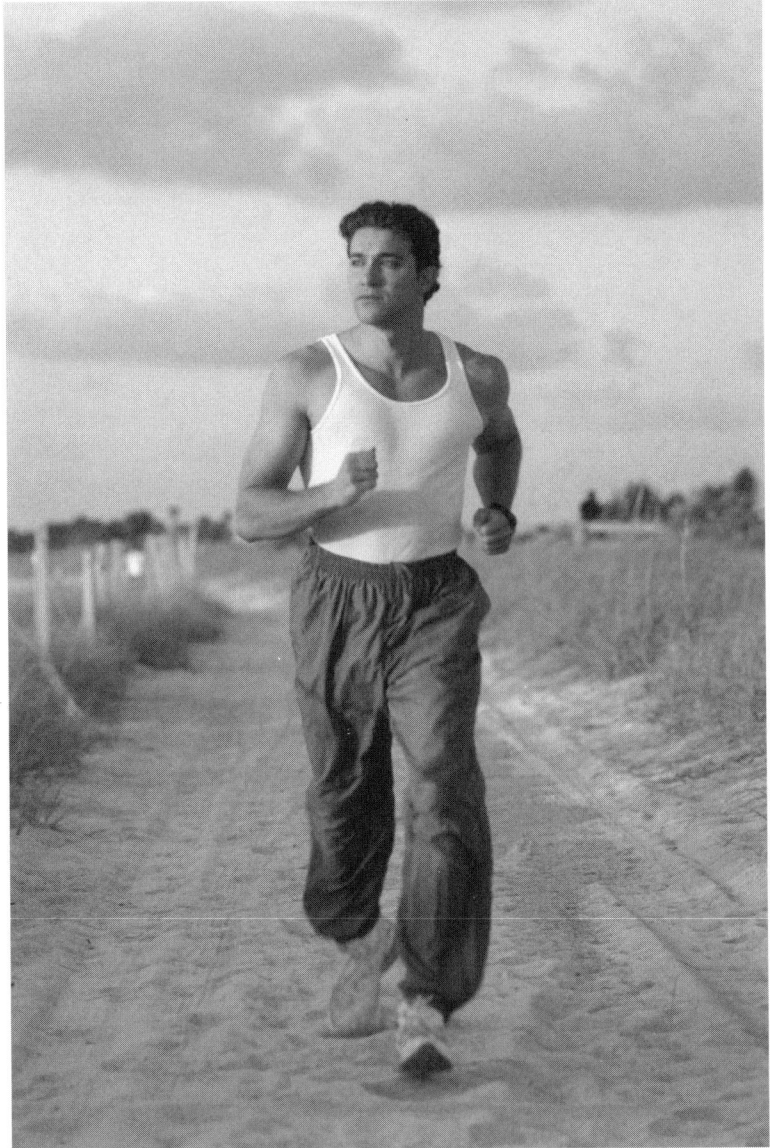

Endorphins are the body's own mood-elevating, pain-relieving compounds. Along with physical benefits, such as improved muscle tone and heart rate, exercise makes people feel better. It also has been shown to improve self-image. Numerous studies have examined the effect of exercise as a mood-elevating therapy and all have indicated positive results.

Today, more than ever, medical and mental health professionals believe that the body and brain are intricately connected. This belief has encouraged physicians, psychiatrists, psychologists, and other therapists to recommend treatments that address a person's physical and emotional needs in hope of finding the most effective relief from depression.

6

Getting Help

THE NUMEROUS TREATMENTS available will not help anyone who believes that depression is nothing more than evidence of a weak will or a poor attitude. Unfortunately, this is the opinion of a great number of people whose medical condition qualifies for a diagnosis of depression. The low self-esteem they feel because of the disease becomes a wall that prevents them from seeking help. The impatient, snap-out-of-it attitude that is widespread in the general public only makes it harder for people with depression to see past that wall. Yet without compassionate help, people with depression often go untreated. They continue to believe they are unworthy of help.

These negative views about depression can be changed in at least three ways. First, people everywhere can learn more and talk more about the disease at home, in the workplace, and during social gatherings. Second, activists can lobby for changes in current insurance coverage, which limits payments for hospital care and prescription drugs for the condition diagnosed as depression. Third, through support groups, depression sufferers can learn about their disease, share their experience and compassion with others, and build networking systems that can lend clout to efforts to secure favorable legal treatment on issues relating to depression.

These great changes must start with individuals, but the mission is not impossible. A similar shift in society's thinking occurred relatively rapidly concerning alcoholism. Not too many years ago, alcoholics were simply considered weak-willed men and women who couldn't stay away from liquor. Now more is known about the disease of alcoholism. Treatment programs are available in almost every city, and support groups are also plentiful. People who acknowledge that they are recovering alcoholics are respected for their effort.

It's been said that for every alcoholic at least ten other lives are affected. Depression has a similar ripple effect. Often caring friends and family are unable to convey to their loved ones the concern that mounts as symptoms of the disease become more alarming. Denial is a major hurdle to overcome with both a person who drinks to excess and a person who has acquired one of the forms of depression.

Many alcoholics think they can control their use of the substance and their behavior. The effects of the substance have clouded their perspective, however. Depressed people already are operating with reduced ability to think clearly,

A mother and son walk together. Supportive family members may be able to encourage a depressed person to seek help.

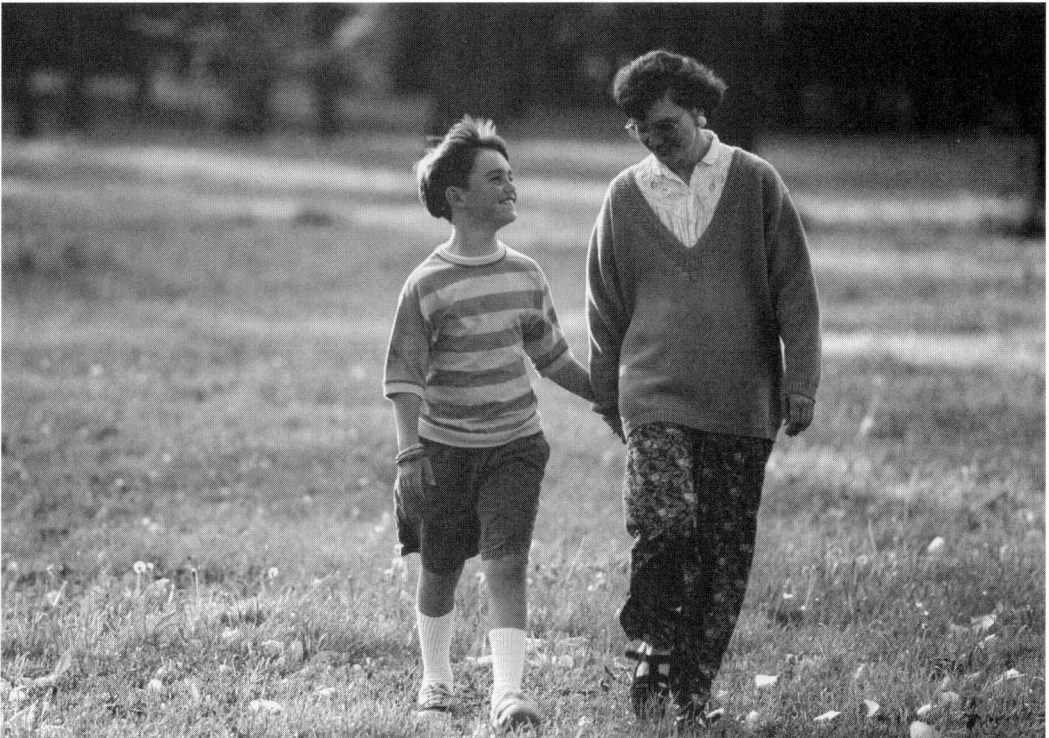

and that condition makes it hard for others to reason with them. Yet if family members despair of persuading a depressed person to seek professional help, their act of giving up almost always compounds the sufferer's feelings of low self-worth and isolation. It is then that the danger of suicide becomes a reality.

The comedian Joan Rivers, an acknowledged depression sufferer, has this to say about going for help:

> You must go for help. You cannot do it yourself when you're that depressed. Even if you go for help and it doesn't seem like it's helping, it's still helping. Part of the help is that someone is there to at least share it with you. Nobody else wants to hear it. When my therapist said, "You're totally correct, everything has fallen apart, your life is a shambles," that was tremendously important in the healing process. Someone gave me the right to feel the way I was feeling.[25]

How family and friends can offer help

It is often difficult to begin to encourage a loved one to seek help, and not knowing what to say may prevent a person who wants to do the right thing from introducing this sensitive subject. No one wants to make a person who is already hurting feel even worse. And potential helpers certainly don't want to increase the paranoid mania that is sometimes associated with bipolar disorders. Yet there are certain approaches that may elicit a favorable response from a person who is depressed.

A Continuum of Intervention Strategies

Treatment Settings Based on Level of Impairment

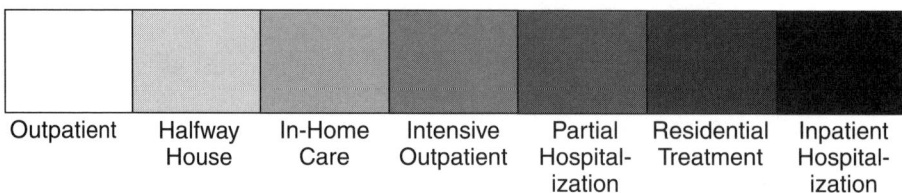

Outpatient	Halfway House	In-Home Care	Intensive Outpatient	Partial Hospitalization	Residential Treatment	Inpatient Hospitalization

A whole array of treatment settings is available to psychiatric patients.

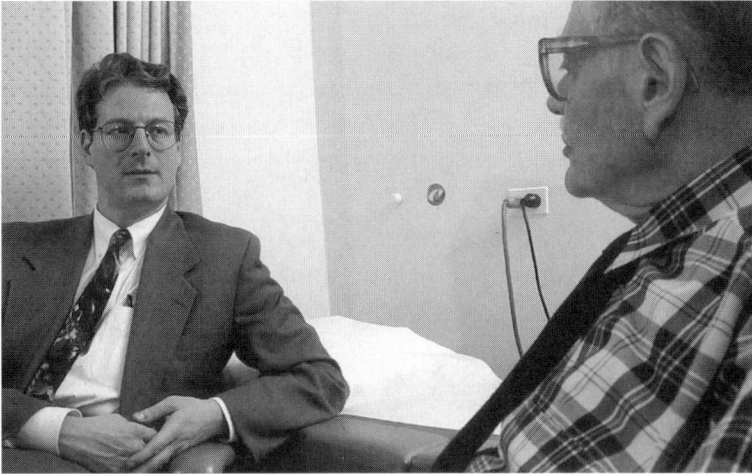

Dr. John A. Rush, a pioneer in the field of treating mental illness, has authored many books about depression. He offers specific tips about talking with sufferers and encouraging them to seek help:

> The best way is to say to them, "Look, I've known you a long time, and you are not yourself. Here's what I see. I talk to you, you break out in tears. You look like you haven't slept in a week. I ask you questions; your mind is not staying on track. I don't think you're doing this on purpose. I think you're ill. I think you have a depression or something is wrong, and you need, in my view, to go get a real expert opinion, not advice from the neighbor and the dog catcher and everybody else, and I'm willing to go with you. I'm willing to make an appointment for you. I don't want to just sit on this thing." [26]

This simple, honest speech might offer the depressed person just the right opening to finally admit all the fear and hurt he or she is feeling. Such an admission is usually the first step in the healing process, and having someone who knows where to go for help is a valuable plus.

A family physician might be a logical choice for that first appointment, although unless he or she is familiar with depressive illness, the trip might be just the beginning. One might also find out whether the community mental health center, the nearby hospitals, or any local university medical center has a special program for treating depression.

People who are showing symptoms of bipolar disorder—not eating or sleeping for days, or experiencing delusions and hallucinations—might need to be admitted to a hospital. These people are in the midst of severe depressive episodes and could be at risk of hurting themselves or others. A person who is seeing things that are not there should not be driving a car or caring for young children.

Without question, any person considering suicide needs immediate attention, preferably from a mental health professional or a physician. Many school counselors and pastors are trained to assist in detecting whether someone might be suicidal and offer prompt guidance regarding treatment.

Living with depression

It is important for those diagnosed with depression, and especially bipolar disorder, to understand that their illness will not go away. The disease will remain under control only with continued treatment; a person may feel better and wish to discontinue treatment, but this is a serious mistake.

Almost everyone who takes an antidepressant sooner or later starts to feel better, and many decide they would like to stop taking the drug. For some, it's a matter of money: a month's supply of one popular drug could run as much as $70. Others hate being dependent on a drug to feel normal. Some would still rather not face the fact that they have a problem they can't handle on their own.

People with depression must be reassured that family and friends understand that the condition results from a biochemical imbalance and can be corrected through medication or psychotherapy, or other treatments. They need to be reminded that these treatments for depression are just as essential as insulin for diabetics and chemotherapy for cancer patients. Psychotherapist Kathryn Foster says she must often emphasize to clients the importance of sticking with their prescribed medication:

> I ask my clients to hold their medication in their hands and say "Thank you, God, that there's a simple way to handle depression." When they start to feel better and want to consider

going off the antidepressant, I ask them to come in and talk to me so we can monitor their feelings and behaviors while they wean off. Because if the symptoms come back, they might not be able to tell the difference, but I will. [27]

The inner struggle over depression is sometimes a powerful obstacle to obtaining professional help. External factors can also weigh against a person suffering from the disease.

Health insurance conflicts

The cost of treatment is one of the external factors that may keep those who need it from seeking professional help. Psychotherapy and antidepressants are not cheap. An average cost for one year's treatment of depression, including medication and therapy sessions, can run close to $3,000. And many insurance companies do not grant depression or other mental health diseases the same status as strictly physical conditions such as diabetes, pregnancy, or a broken bone. Thus coverage for mental health benefits is often much lower than the coverage available for the more traditional medical categories.

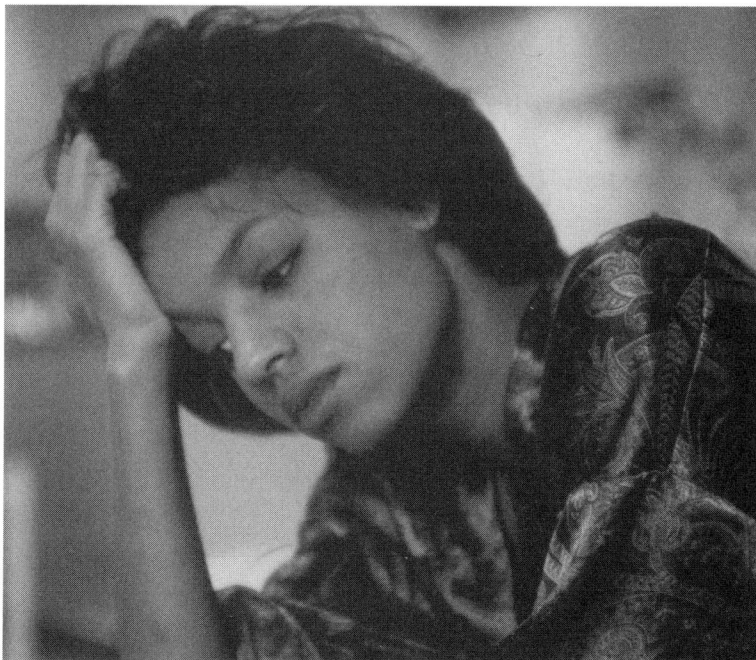

Some people avoid seeking help because their insurance companies will not pay for conventional treatments for depression.

Dr. Lewis Judd, chairman of the Department of Psychiatry at the University of California, has studied the cost of depression and how the disease affects society. He believes greater acceptance of depression as a medical illness will lead to more awareness among the general public, the workforce, and the insurance companies:

> We calculated that depression is costing San Diego alone, each year, $200 million. [People in the work force] are not being treated, are disabled, and suffering and dysfunctional from depression, and [the companies] don't even know about it. We can demonstrate that appropriate treatment and early recognition could save enormous amounts of money for corporations. . . .
>
> At a time when we know more about depression than ever, at a time when we can diagnose it reliably and treat it successfully, it's ironic that the options for people getting treatment are increasingly remote and difficult. The trend in the insurance industry is to exclude more and more and to have fewer and fewer benefits for mental disorders like depression.[28]

Even for those who lack health insurance coverage for their disease, there is some help available. Organized support groups are among the most accessible means of dealing with depression.

Support groups

Support groups help people reduce feelings of isolation, one of the most common problems resulting from depression. In support groups, people discuss experiences and feelings they sometimes have trouble sharing with friends and family members who have not had to deal with depression except as observers.

Studies done in the 1970s showed that social isolation releases the so-called stress hormones and can actually trigger depressive feelings. When people interacted with one another and talked about their feelings, the levels of these hormones decreased. Experts now believe that social contact helps dam the flood of stress hormones. Edward Madara, director of the American Self-Help Clearinghouse, believes that support groups offer a healthy atmosphere in which participants may discuss their particular problems:

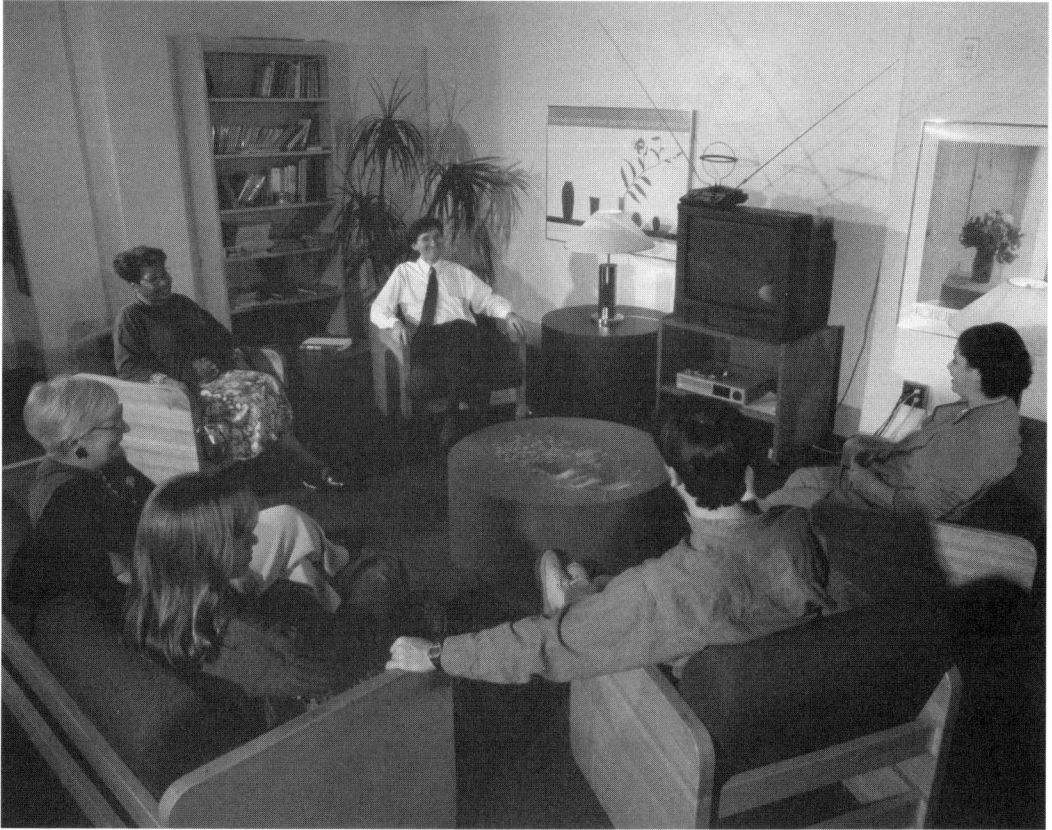

A group of depressed individuals form a support group to help one another.

When you sit down with others who have shared your experience—no matter whether it's depression, diabetes, multiple sclerosis, or an unfaithful spouse—you feel a sense of comfort and closeness no professional relationship can match.[29]

Support groups can help people suffering from depression make a smoother transition from immediate treatment into the long-term acceptance of their disease. This support enhances their feelings of self-worth, too. Support groups can also offer resources such as psychiatrist and psychotherapist recommendations, as well as current information about controversial treatments and self-care tips. In the past, support groups have even helped change laws and public opinion. However, their greatest strength is in serving as a major forum for the relief of stress and the building up of each person's self-esteem.

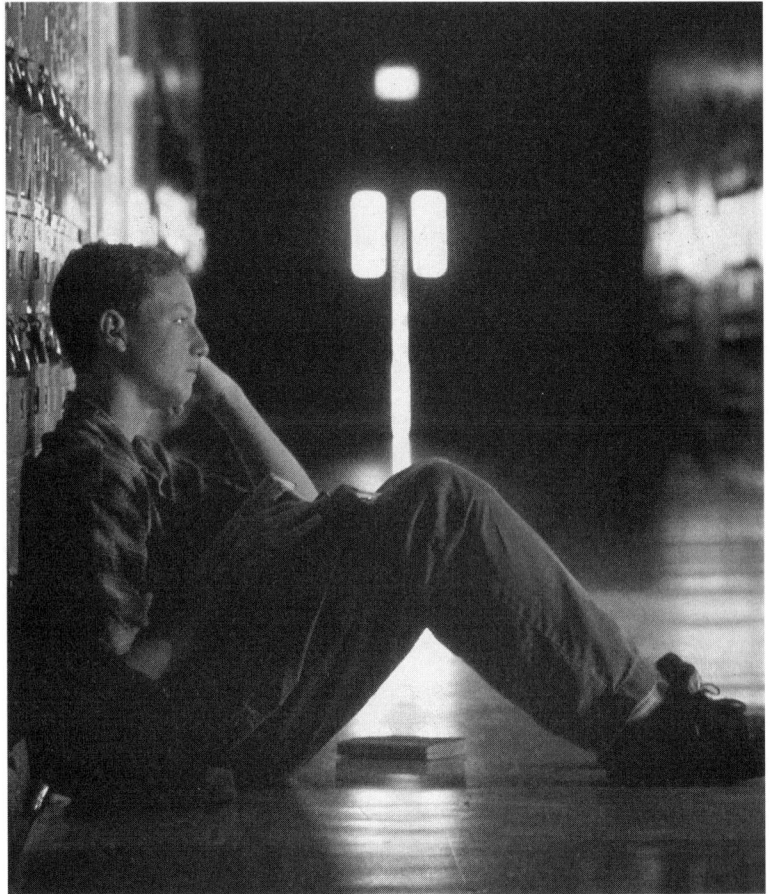

Depression is almost always treatable. In order to eliminate the disease, people must learn to recognize the symptoms and seek help.

Anyone suffering from depression who enters a support group meeting is an instant peer. Every person in the room can relate to the newcomer's feelings of choking despair and suffocating loneliness. Everyone understands the feelings a depressed person may have thought were his or hers alone. As members gain emotional strength, they in turn offer support to the newer members, increasing their own feelings of self-worth. Not only are they feeling healthier, they are also making a contribution, which is another essential part of the healing process.

The only barrier left

Today the only barrier between suffering with depression and enjoying health is failure to recognize the symptoms and to know them for what they are: signs of a biochemical imbalance. If such informed broad-mindedness had been prevalent earlier in this century, perhaps Winston Churchill, a man of outstanding political contributions, who also felt unworthy because of chronic depression, would have received help. Perhaps he could have believed what the rest of the world well knew—that in addition to being one of the greatest leaders of the century, he was also a worthy individual.

Notes

Introduction

1. Quoted in Kathy Cronkite, *On the Edge of Darkness.* New York: Delta, 1995, p. 2.
2. Quoted in Cronkite, *On the Edge of Darkness,* p. 72.

Chapter 1: About Depression

3. Quoted in Cronkite, *On the Edge of Darkness,* p. 20.
4. David Hughes, interview with author, Joshua, TX, February 15, 1997.
5. Quoted in Jean Block, "My Moods Were Out of Control," *Good Housekeeping,* April 1997, pp. 80–84.
6. Quoted in Carol Turkington, *Making the Prozac Decision.* Los Angeles: Lowell House, 1995, p. 7.
7. John C. Markowitz, "Depression," *New York Times Syndicate,* December 2, 1996, pp. 1–2. http://nytsyn.com/live/ Depression/337_1202096_150028_11498.html

Chapter 2: What Causes Depression?

8. Quoted in Wayne Drevets, "Missing Cells Tied to Depression," *Detroit News,* October 27, 1997.

Chapter 3: Those at Risk

9. Kathryn Foster, interview with author, Fort Worth, TX, February 24, 1998.
10. Mark S. Gold, *Good News About Depression.* New York: Villard Books, 1997, p. 276.
11. Gold, *Good News About Depression,* p. 281.
12. Gold, *Good News About Depression,* p. 290.
13. Marguerite Parke, interview with author, Crowley, TX, January 5, 1998.

14. Quoted in Colette Dowling, *You Mean I Don't Have to Feel This Way? New Help for Depression, Anxiety, and Addiction.* New York: Charles Scribner's Sons, 1991, p. 128.

Chapter 4: Treating Depression

15. Gold, *Good News About Depression,* p. 242.
16. Quoted in Turkington, *Making the Prozac Decision,* p. 2.
17. Foster, interview.
18. Quoted in Ricki Lewis, "Evening Out the Ups and Downs of Manic-Depressive Illness," *FDA Consumer,* June 1996, p. 28.
19. Quoted in Cronkite, *On the Edge of Darkness,* p. 181.

Chapter 5: Alternative Treatments

20. Quoted in Sandra G. Boodman, "Shock Therapy . . . It's Back," *Washington Post,* September 24, 1996, p. Z14.
21. Quoted in Cronkite, *On The Edge of Darkness,* p. 289.
22. Norman E. Rosenthal, *Winter Blues.* New York: Guilford Press, 1993, p. 257.
23. Zoltan P. Rona, "Depression," *HealthLink Articles,* March 14, 1998, p. 1. http://www.selene.com/healthlink/dep.html
24. Herbert Benson, "The Relaxation Response," in Daniel Goelman and Joel Gurin, eds., *Mind–Body Medicine.* New York: Consumer Books, 1993, p. 250.

Chapter 6: Getting Help

25. Quoted in Cronkite, *On the Edge of Darkness,* p. 310.
26. Quoted in Cronkite, *On the Edge of Darkness,* p. 219.
27. Foster, interview.
28. Quoted in Cronkite, *On the Edge of Darkness,* pp. 317–18.
29. Quoted in "Support Groups," *Depression.com,* March 12, 1998, p. 1. http://www.depression.com/anti/anti/_25_support.htm

Glossary

anorexia: An eating disorder marked by extreme weight loss, often causing secondary malnutrition and hormonal changes.

antidepressant: A prescription medication designed to help alleviate depression.

aromatherapy: A mood-elevating therapy using essential oils from plants.

behavioral therapy: Psychological counseling that focuses on changing behavior.

bipolar disorder: Extreme depression characterized by alternating high and low mood swings; can be accompanied by hallucinations or delusions.

bulimia: An eating disorder marked by frequent episodes of overeating followed immediately by purging.

chronic: A persisting condition.

cognitive therapy: Psychological counseling that focuses on changing the way a person thinks about oneself.

depression: A biochemical disorder marked by sadness, inactivity, difficulty in thinking and concentration, a significant increase or decrease in appetite and time spent sleeping, feelings of dejection and hopelessness, and sometimes suicidal tendencies.

dopamine: A chemical neurotransmitter thought to play a role in concentration and control of motor and cognitive impulses.

eating disorders: Emotional disorders in which a person's abuse of food is a symptom of an underlying psychological problem.

electroconvulsive therapy (ECT): A treatment for depression involving the use of electricity in small pulses to cause convulsions in the brain and alter chemical imbalances.

ginkgo: An herb studied for its success in neutralizing neurotransmitter levels in depression sufferers.

hormone: A substance that affects growth and proper development in living things.

hyperthyroidism: A condition in which the thyroid gland is overactive.

hypothyroidism: A condition in which the thyroid gland is underactive.

interpersonal therapy: Psychological counseling that helps people analyze how they interact with others.

learned response: A habitual reaction to chronic stressful or traumatic events.

major depression: A form of depression marked by feelings of hopelessness, irritability, difficulty with concentration, and suicidal thoughts.

mania: Mental disorder characterized by extreme enthusiasm, excitement, or passion and sometimes delusions, restlessness, or risk-taking behavior.

melatonin: Brain chemical necessary for proper growth and development.

mood-elevating therapies: Nontraditional treatments focusing on lifting mood.

neurotransmitter: Chemical substance that carries impulses from one nerve cell to another.

norepinephrine: Powerful neurotransmitter known to affect several body functions as well as concentration and focus.

pellagra: Disease caused by a vitamin deficiency. Symptoms can include stomach discomfort and delirium, hallucinations and eventual dementia.

phototherapy: Treatment for depression that uses light to increase levels of melatonin.

postpartum: The time period immediately following birth.

premenstrual syndrome (PMS): A condition affecting some women a few days before menstruation. Common symptoms include bloating, severe mood swings, and headaches.

psychotherapy: Counseling using cognitive, behavioral, or interpersonal therapy, or some combination of these.

seasonal affective disorder (SAD): Emotional disorder marked by low mood and energy affecting many people during fall and winter.

serotonin: Neurotransmitter believed to be necessary for proper motor and cognitive control; low levels have been tied to depression.

St. John's wort: An herb that has been found useful in treating some depression.

traumatic: Extremely stressful.

unipolar disorder: Another term for major depression.

Organizations
to Contact

American Psychiatric Association
1400 K St. NW
Washington, DC 20005
(202) 797-4900

An organization of psychiatric professionals.

American Self-Help Clearinghouse
St. Clares Riverside Medical Center
Danville, NJ 07834
(973) 625-7101

Nonprofit organization that keeps track of nearly 700 support groups in the United States and directs people to local groups that can meet their specific needs.

D/ART DEPRESSION: Awareness, Recognition and Treatment
5600 Fishers Lane
Rockville, MD 20857
(301) 443-3877

A program of the federal government to educate the public, primary care providers, and mental health specialists about depressive illnesses.

National Alliance for the Mentally Ill
200 North Glebe Rd., Suite 501
Arlington, VA 22203-3754
(703) 524-7600

Nationwide chapters offer support, publications, information, and a toll-free help line: (800) 950-NAMI (6264).

National Coalition for the Mentally Ill in the
  Criminal Justice System
2470 Westlake Ave. North, Suite 101
Seattle, WA 98109
(206) 285-7422

This organization helps the mentally ill and their families
when they become involved in the criminal justice system.

National Foundation for Depressive Illness
PO Box 2257
New York, NY 10116
(212) 268-4260; (800) 248-4344

This group seeks to educate the public about depressive illness, its consequences, and treatability. Provides information
and referrals to physicians and other professionals.

National Institutes of Mental Health
5600 Fishers Lane
Rockville, MD 20857
(301) 443-3877

Part of the U.S. Public Health Service, which provides information and additional sources regarding mental illnesses of
all types.

National Mental Health Association
1021 Prince St.
Alexandria, VA 22314-2971
(710) 684-7722; (800) 248-4344

An eighty-year-old voluntary charitable organization that ad-
dresses mental health needs of communities, states, and the
nation through outreach and referral programs.

NOSAD

PO Box 40190

Washington, DC 20016

This self-help group for people with seasonal affective disorder (SAD) provides a newsletter and support for patients and their families.

SADA

PO Box 989

London SW72PZ

A United Kingdom registered charity that organizes meetings for sufferers of SAD and professionals. SADA provides a network of information and support groups.

Suggestions for Further Reading

Aaron T. Beck, *Depression.* Philadelphia: University of Pennsylvania Press, 1996. A comprehensive overview of depression, its symptoms, and treatments.

David D. Burns, *Feeling Good: The New Mood Therapy.* New York: William Morrow, 1980. A clinically proven treatment for depression from the University of Pennsylvania School of Medicine.

Robert M. Giller, *Natural Prescriptions: Dr. Giller's Natural Treatments and Vitamin Therapies for Over 100 Common Ailments.* New York: Ballantine, 1995. An up-to-date guide combining years of medical practice involving natural treatments.

Bill Gottlieb, *New Choices in Natural Healing.* Emmaus, PA: Rodale Press, 1997. Listing of over 1,800 of the best self-help remedies from the world of alternative medicine.

Francis Mark Mondimore, *Depression: The Mood Disease.* Baltimore: Johns Hopkins University Press, 1993. An easy-to-understand look at depression, case studies, and treatment plans.

Arthur and Irma Myers, *Why You Feel Down and What You Can Do About It.* New York: Charles Scribner's Sons, 1982. Straight talk for teens about depression and its physical, emotional, and intellectual signs.

John Preston, *You Can Beat Depression.* San Luis Obispo, CA: Impact Publishers, 1989. A practical guide for recognizing depression and overcoming the disease.

Sandra Salmans, *Depression: Questions You Have . . . Answers You Need.* Allentown, PA: People's Medical Society, 1995. The most common questions regarding depression, its symptoms, and treatments.

Julia Thorne, *You Are Not Alone.* New York: Harper Perennial, 1993. Compilation of various people's accounts of their depressive illnesses and the effects of the disease on their lives.

Elizabeth Wurtzel, *Prozac Nation.* New York: Riverhead Books, 1995. A raw look from the inside of a woman's depression and the struggles she encountered.

Works Consulted

Herbert Benson, "The Relaxation Response," in Daniel Goelman and Joel Gurin, eds., *Mind–Body Medicine.* New York: Consumer Books, 1993.

Jean Block, "My Moods Were Out of Control," *Good Housekeeping,* April 1997.

Sandra Boodman, "Shock Therapy . . . It's Back," *Washington Post,* September 24, 1996, p. Z14.

Edwin Cassem and Joseph T. Coyle, "Depression," *The Harvard Mahoney Neuroscience Institute Letter,* Special Issue, 1998. http://www.med.harvard.edu/publication/On_The_Brain/Volume 2/Special/SpDepr.html

Jeff Cohen and Norman Soloman, "Psychiatric Technique Gets Shocking Boost from Media," *Psych Central: Dr. John Grohol's Mental Health Page,* 1995. http://www.grohol.com/electro.htm

Kathy Cronkite, *On the Edge of Darkness.* New York: Delta, 1995.

Debra Deren, "Children and Depression," *Wings of Depression,* February 17, 1998. http://members.aol.com/depress/children.htm#causes

Colette Dowling, *You Mean I Don't Have to Feel This Way? New Help for Depression, Anxiety, and Addiction.* New York: Charles Scribner's Sons, 1991.

Wayne Drevets, "Missing Cells Tied to Depression," *Detroit News,* October 27, 1997.

Barbara Fitzsimmons, "Mood for Thought," *San Diego Union Tribune,* December 9, 1996.

Michael Gitlin, "Bipolar Disorders: Clinical Complexities, Current Challenges," *The Journal.* Vol. 6, Issue 2, 1998.

Susan Godbey and Rachelle Schaaf, "Sad Habit," *Prevention,* August 1997.

Mark Gold, *Good News About Depression.* New York: Villard, 1997.

Ivan Goldberg, *Questions and Answers About Depression and Its Treatment.* Philadelphia: The Charles Press, 1993.

John Griest, *Depression and Its Treatment.* Washington, DC: American Psychiatric Press, 1984.

Steven Hollon, "Ask the Experts," *Scientific American,* January 22, 1998. http://www.sciam.com/askexpert/medicine/medicine1/html

Jackie Robert Kelley II, "Learning to Conquer My Demons," *Essence,* May 1997.

Kenneth Kendler, Ellen Waltere, and Kim Truett, "Heredity vs. Environment in Depression," *The Harvard Mental Health Letter,* July 1995.

Peter Kramer, *Listening to Prozac.* New York: Viking, 1993.

Ricki Lewis, "Evening Out the Ups and Downs of Manic-Depressive Illness," *FDA Consumer,* June 1996.

John Mann, "Nature Medicine," *Thrive Health News,* December 30, 1997.

John Markowitz, "Depression," *New York Times Syndicate,* December 2, 1996. http://nytsyn.com/live/Depression/337_1202096_150028_11498.html

Sue Miller, "A Natural Mood Booster," *Newsweek,* May 5, 1997.

Mary Pinkowish, "Treating Depression: Little Touches Count," *Patient Care,* December 15, 1996.

Joel Robertson, *Natural Prozac.* San Francisco: HarperCollins, 1997.

Zoltan P. Rona, "Depression," *HealthLink Articles,* March 14, 1998. http://www.selene.com/healthlink/dep.html

Norman Rosenthal, *Winter Blues.* New York: Guilford Press, 1993.

Melvin Saunders, "Self-Healing and Your 100% Brain," *Alternative Heal for the 21st Century,* March 12, 1998. http://www.tiac.net/users/seeker/selfheal.html

Michael Stone, *The Borderline Syndromes.* New York: McGraw-Hill, 1980.

Jamie Talan, "Shock Therapy," *Newsday,* April 10, 1990.

Carol Turkington, *Making the Prozac Decision.* Los Angeles: Lowell House, 1995.

Index

Picture Credits

About the Author

Robyn M. Weaver is a writer, editor, and Continuing Education instructor at Texas Christian University. She travels across the country, leading seminars about the mechanics of writing and also giving workshops on how to use writing exercises to help heal emotional wounds.